CANCER ETIOLOGY, DIAGNOSIS AND TREATMENTS

GASTRIC PERITONEAL CARCINOMATOSIS

PRINCIPLES OF SURGERY AND TREATMENT OPTIONS

CANCER ETIOLOGY, DIAGNOSIS AND TREATMENTS

Additional books and e-books in this series can be found on Nova's website under the Series tab.

SURGERY - PROCEDURES, COMPLICATIONS, AND RESULTS

Additional books and e-books in this series can be found on Nova's website under the Series tab.

CANCER ETIOLOGY, DIAGNOSIS AND TREATMENTS

GASTRIC PERITONEAL CARCINOMATOSIS

PRINCIPLES OF SURGERY AND TREATMENT OPTIONS

FERNANDO LÓPEZ MOZOS
AND
ROBERTO MARTÍ OBIOL
EDITORS

nova
Medicine & Health
New York

NOTICE TO THE READER

Library of Congress Cataloging-in-Publication Data

ISBN: 978-1-53619-487-6

Published by Nova Science Publishers, Inc. † New York

CONTENTS

FOREWORD

"If you think medical innovation is expensive, try disease"
- Mary Woodard Lasker

The cost of healthcare in the United States of America (US) is significant. According to the World Bank, the US spends 17.9% of Gross Domestic Product on health. This is up from 15.6% just ten years ago. Given an aging cadre of baby boomers and strong correlation between age and healthcare expenditures, the proportion of GDP spent on healthcare is likely to continue rising. For example, given current trends, the number of Americans with Alzheimer's disease is expected to grow to 13.5 million and cost the US $20 trillion by 2050, according to the Alzheimer's Association. Given these projections, a number of policymakers and politicians in the US have focused on the healthcare expenditure issue, and this reflects the thinking of the populace. Polls conducted by Harris Research showed that 44% of US adults are "extremely worried" or "very worried" about paying for rising health-care costs.

Policymakers generally discuss three ways to address the growing healthcare expenditure problem: (1) cut back on spending, either by limiting the amount paid for products and services, or by reducing the level of products and services being offered; (2) continue on the current path, which likely means continued increases in spending and thus, the raising of funds to support that spending through increased taxation, insurance premiums, or borrowing, (3) maintain services but limit spending increases by eliminating waste and improving efficiency. While this is a desirable option, finding efficiencies has an upper limit and may not address the full scale of the problem.

There is a fourth option for limiting healthcare cost increases: Research and Innovation – in essence, the discovery of more cures for disease. Historical "definitive cures" that prevent disease (e.g., vaccines which have successfully eliminated polio from the US and much of the world. Vaccines are the most potent weapons against the spread of most infectious diseases, and will provide the solution to ending the current pandemic of SARS-CoV-2. Some cures eliminate the impact of a disease after it has taken hold (e.g., insulin for Type I diabetes) have, and will continue to save the US economy billions of dollars every year. The up-front investment in basic research to understand disease processes, and applied research to intervene effectively in that process to cure the disease, is significant. While the discovery of a cure (i.e., the return) is not guaranteed, only by allocating significant resources toward the cause and distributing those resources effectively, can we have any hope of future breakthroughs. Given past experience, the potential return on those breakthroughs is staggering. Even more, the analyses included in this volume suggest that preventive measures such as daily exercise and changes in diet can provide a virtually infinite return on investment and have an impact across multiple health domains with essentially no unwanted side effects. Now, it is up to scientists to carry out research that will provide insights into why so few Americans follow these behavioral guidelines, and help policymakers change this reality.

The US is one of only a few nations on earth with the ability to invest in the level of research that is necessary to make significant advancements in cures. First, it has the economic capacity to invest the necessary resources up-front, wherein the return on investment might be decades in the future. Second, it has a well-established education system and research base to ramp up the necessary research activity quickly. Finally, it has the culture of innovation and outside-of-the-box thinking that is so critical for cures breakthroughs. All that is needed is the cultural and political will.

This volume provides a policy foundation for cures discovery by examining the burden of illness, economic impact of past cures, and potential economic impact of future cures across multiple diseases and disease categories. The diseases included in this volume were selected because many of them represent a significant burden and economic impact in the US (i.e., cardiovascular disease, diabetes) and/or the world (i.e., malaria). It examines the [economic] returns across a wide spectrum of disease categories, using a common frame of reference. Where cures have already been discovered and implemented, such as the polio vaccine, an historical analysis is provided that estimates the human and economic impact of the disease prior to the introduction of the cure. The total impact of the disease if the cure had not been discovered as well as an estimate of the ongoing future annual cost of the disease without the cure, is presented. Where cures are nonexistent or limited, such as Alzheimer's disease, estimates of the human impact and burden of disease, as well as the overall economic cost of the discase to the US, is presented. This provides an estimate of the potential costs savings to be achieved with the development of a cure.

By examining the economic impact of these different highly burdensome diseases, and the cures that have been discovered to ameliorate that impact, this volume provides insight into the cures process and project future potential economic impact of cures on the health system in the US and around the world. This will allow policymakers to make informed decisions regarding how much to invest in cures. As such, this volume is a key summary of the economics of diseases and their cures.

Calum Macpherson, PhD, DIC, MEVPC, FRSPH, FSB
Dean of Graduate Studies and Director of Research,
St. George's University
Director, Windward Islands Research and Education Foundation
(WINDREF)

ACKNOWLEDGMENTS

Thanks to *Mercé V Electromedicina S.L* for their support during these years.

In: Gastric Peritoneal Carcinomatosis ISBN: 978-1-53619-487-6
Editors: F. López Mozos et al.

Chapter 1

EPIDEMIOLOGY OF GASTRIC CANCER

Rosa Martí Fernández*, MD, Roberto Martí Obiol, PhD and Fernando López Mozos, PhD

Esophagogastric and Peritoneal Oncology Surgery Unit
Department of Surgery
Hospital Clínico Universitario, Valencia, Spain

ABSTRACT

Gastric cancer remains a common cause of cancer mortality throughout the world, with great geographic variability in its distribution. Due to the absence of specific symptoms, it is usually diagnosed in advanced stages in most countries, where there are no early detection programs. Up to 60% of patients are diagnosed in advanced stages. Furthermore, the natural history of the tumor is spread to the peritoneum, liver, and lung. The peritoneal spread of gastric cancer is favored by a number of factors specific to the tumor, the patient, or secondary to primary resection surgery. Among tumor-specific factors, genetic alterations have been described to favor the growth of cells detached from the tumor in the peritoneum. An early diagnosis of the disease is essential for a better treatment of peritoneal carcinomatosis of gastric origin.

* Corresponding Author's E-mail: rosamartifernandez@gmail.com.

Computed tomography and laparoscopy are the mainstays of diagnosis. Once the diagnosis of peritoneal carcinomatosis has been established, we have several treatment options that include chemotherapy and surgical treatment, either alone or in combination with chemotherapy.

INTRODUCTION

Gastric cancer is the fifth most common cancer worldwide, accounting for 5.7% of all cancers. However, it represents the third leading cause of cancer death, being responsible for almost 800,000 deaths/year[1,2]. It presents a wide geographic variation with its maximum representation in Asian countries, mainly Korea, China and Japan, and regions where its incidence decreases drastically, the United States and Africa.

There are a series of risk factors associated with the development of gastric cancer:

- Genetic factors
- Helicobacter pylori
- Epstein-Barr virus
- Race and gender
- Smoking
- Diet: salt, alcohol, nitrites
- Socioeconomic status
- Blood group
- Obesity
- Previous gastric surgery
- Pernicious anemia
- Radiation

Due to the absence of screening, with the exception of Southeast Asian countries where it is performed by biennial upper digestive endoscopy from the age of 50, the diagnosis is usually made in advanced stages with a low probability of achieving curative treatment. The main sites of tumor spread are the liver, lung, and peritoneum. Thus, up to 60% of patients are diagnosed at an advanced stage, with little or no capacity to achieve effective treatment. Up to 14% of patients will present with synchronous carcinomatosis at the time of diagnosis [3], while 15-52% will develop it during postoperative follow-up [4]. The appearance of peritoneal metastases, either during follow-up or synchronously with the diagnosis of the primary gastric neoplasia, leads to survival rates that did not exceed 3-4 months in the past in most series [4, 5] .

These high rates of recurrence in the form of peritoneal metastases after surgery have two possible explanations. One of them is that tumor cell dissemination occurs during the manipulation of the primary tumor, particularly when the serous layer is involved. Another is the dissemination produced as a consequence of some aspects of the surgical procedure:

- from sectioned lymphatic vessels
- blood remains contaminated with tumor cells
- tumor margins affected or close to the edge of surgical resection

The process of celomic dissemination in the peritoneum requires a series of processes that involve different genetic alterations in order to achieve the detachment of cancer cells from the tumor and produce a seeding on the peritoneal surface. The procedure begins with the shedding of cells from the tumor, after surgery or spontaneously, by down-regulation of intercellular adhesion processes that involve some molecules such as E-cadherin. Subsequently, the cells enter the peritoneum due to the expression of adhesion factors, such as CD44. Finally, tumor cells secrete vascular endothelial growth factor (VEGF), favoring angiogenesis and tumor proliferation, forming carcinomatous nodules [6-10]. Besides, the malignant cells are covered by a fibrinous exudate that protect them from chemotherapic agents administered intravenously being only susceptible to HIPEC regimens. This process is known as tumor cell entrapment.

Recently, it has been reported four molecular subtypes of gastric cancer that confer different probability of progression and different prognostic. These are: MSS/TP53 + MSS/TP53 - MSI and MSS/EMT [11].

There is an intense correlation between the expression of HIF-1α and the development of peritoneal carcinomatosis in cases of gastric cancer [12].

Nowadays a series of risk factors have been described for the development of peritoneal carcinomatosis [4,13,14]. J Li et al. have developed a scale to classify patients into risk groups. Through the completion of the Gastric cancer peritoneal carcinomatosis score (GCPS) we can classify patients in different risk groups and design an appropriate follow-up for each patient according to the risk of recurrence. However, there is no evidence that intensive follow-up of high-risk patients increases survival [4].

Table 1. Gastric cancer peritoneal carcinomatosis score (GCPS)

Patient and tumor characteristics	Score
Age (years)	
18-39 years versus 60+	6
40-59 years versus 60+	3
60+	0
Race/ethnicity	
Non-Hispanic white	0
Asian/other	0.5
Non-Hispanic black	3
Hispanic	2.5
Clinical T stage	
T1	0
T2	1
T3	1
T4	5.5
Histology	
Intestinal	0
NOS	1
Mucinous	1.5
Diffuse	2.5
Signet ring	3.5
Tumor location	
Proximal	0
Body	2.5
Distal	2.5
Overlapping	4
Tumor grade	
Well-differentiated	0
Moderately well-differentiated	2
Poorly differentiated or undifferentiated	4

NOS: not otherwise specified

Score	%
0-10	3.2
10.5-14	9.5
14.5-17	15
17.5-20	26.1
20-26	46.4

From: Ji L, Selleck MJ, Morgan JW, Wu J, Babcock BD, Shavlik D, et al. Gastric cancer peritoneal carcinomatosis risk score. Ann SurgOncol. 2020;27:240-247.

The diagnosis of peritoneal metastases is a challenge on some occasions since imaging tests, on certain occasions, are not capable to detect all peritoneal involvement. Therefore, the calculation of the peritoneal carcinomatosis index (PCI) may be underestimated preoperatively. Imaging techniques will allow us to identify patients with metastatic disease outside the abdominal cavity, who will not be candidates for cytorreduction and Hyperthermic Intraperitoneal Chemotherapy (HIPEC). Among the diagnostic modalities available, the most widely used are the computed tomography (CT) and the 18F-fluorodeoxyglucose (FDG) positron emission tomography (PET) scan [15]. Another useful tool, and maybe the best for estimating preoperative PCI, is exploratory laparoscopy. This has the advantages of allowing the entire abdominal cavity to be visualized and letting a more precise calculation of the PCI, it allows taking cytology of the ascites fluid as well as determining the presence of biomarkers in peritoneal lavage, which increases the sensitivity in the diagnosis, and this is also a procedure with a low rate of complications [16].

However, in high-risk patients we must not forget the dissemination by the hematic and lymphatic routes, as therefore, in these patients the treatment should not be only locoregional, but also systemic using different chemotherapeutic agents with the aim of completely eradicating the disease. Thus, chemotherapy can have different roles depending on the stage of the patient. Therefore, there are currently different possibilities in the treatment of advanced gastric cancer ranging from traditional treatments with chemotherapy drugs associated or not with radiotherapy to more recently developed treatments such as immunotherapy, total neoadjuvant therapy, gene therapies or nanoparticle therapies [17-20].

For the local treatment of peritoneal carcinomatosis from gastric origin we dispose of multiple possibilities:

- cytoreduction + HIPEC / early Postoperative Intraperitoneal Chemotherapy (EPIC) / Normothermic Intraperitoneal Chemotherapy (NIPEC)
- induction chemotherapy followed of surgery ± HIPEC

- bidirectional chemotherapy and surgery
- Pressured IntraperitonealAreosol Chemotherapy (PIPAC) as induction therapy previous to surgery

Blood-peritoneal barrier conditions that only 3% of the chemotherapy administered intravenously is detected on peritoneal surface. Therefore, the main advantage of the intraperitoneal administration of the chemotherapy, HIPEC or EPIC, is that higher concentration in the peritoneum are achieved compared to systemic administration. When it is applied during the perioperative period and after surgical resection of all visible disease (complete cytorreduction), it has an effect on the possible small amount of disease that remains and before metastatic implants nest between fibrin deposits [21].

Currently, all patients are managed by a multidisciplinary tumor board (MDT) and surgery for carcinomatosis in gastric cancer by cytoreduction and HIPEC is possible in selected patients, with promising results (survival after complete cytorreduction of 18.8 months) [22]. The MDT must be composed by a group of experts in gastric cancer, both medical and surgical specialists, who periodically review each patient in detail in order to select the appropriate treatment for each one. Treatment of these patients should be carried out in high-volume centers and highly specialized units in order to obtain the best results. Preoperative prehabilitation of the patient is essential, which include procedures such as preoperative respiratory physiotherapy, psychological preparation or perioperative immunonutrition, among others, with the aim of improving results [23-25].

The main premise for obtaining good survival results is to achieve a Completeness of Cytoreduction Score (CC) of 0. It has been observed that the addition of HIPEC during surgery has better results in terms of survival, without increasing morbidity, and with 3-year and 5-year recurrence rates of 20.4% and 17.05% versus 5.87% and 3.76%, respectively [22].

HIPEC therapy in gastric cancer can be used in two main ways; prophylaxis against peritoneal carcinomatosis after surgery of a localized primary tumor or as additional therapy during surgery of peritoneal carcinomatosis combined with cytoreduction surgery of all macroscopic disease. The use of HIPEC as a prophylactic therapy has been widely studied in Asia [26,27] demonstrating its effect on survival in patients with serosal invasion or positive lymph nodes, achieving overall 5-year survival rates of 61% in patients treated with HIPEC plus gastrectomy plus lymphadenectomy compared to 42% in patients treated only with surgery [26]. A recent metanalysis proves that surgery and HIPEC administered as prophylactic therapies is safe, does not increase mortality and may prevent peritoneal recurrence in patients without evident metastases and negative cytology [28]. Furthermore, a decreased incidence of peritoneal spread has also been demonstrated in patients receiving HIPEC as a prophylactic therapy. GASTRICHIP trial is a prospective, randomized multicenter phase III clinical study, conducted in Europe, which purpose is to evaluate the effect of prophylactic HIPEC with oxaliplatin in patients with tumors involving the serosa and/or lymph node involvement and/or with positive cytology at peritoncal washing, treated with perioperative systemic chemotherapy and D1-D2 curative gastrectomy [29]. We are expecting the final results in order to confirm if HIPEC is safe and effective in western population preventing peritoneal spread in high risk tumours.

REFERENCES

[1] Shah MA, Kelsen DP. Gastric cancer: A primer on the epidemiology and biology of the disease and an overview of the medical management of advanced disease. *J. Natl.Compr. Canc.Netw.* 2010;8:437-47.

[2] American Joint Committee on Cancer. Stomach. In: *AJCC Cancer Staging Manual*. 8thed. New York, NY: Springer; 2017:203.

[3] Thomassen I R. van Gestel Y, van Ramshorst B D. Luyer M, Bosscha K W. Nienhuijs S et al. Peritoneal carcinomatosis of gastric origin: A population-based study on incidence, survival and risk factors. *Int. J. Cancer*: 134, 622-628 (2014).

[4] Ji L, Selleck MJ, Morgan JW, Xu J, Babcock BD, Shavlik D, Wall NR, Langridge WH, Lum SS, Garberoglio CA, Reeves ME, Solomon N, Namm JP, Senthil M. Gastric Cancer Peritoneal Carcinomatosis Risk Score. *Ann. Surg. Oncol.* 2020 Jan;27(1):240-247. doi: 10.1245/s10434-019-07624-0. *Epub* 2019 Jul 25. PMID: 31346896; PMCID: PMC6925067.

[5] Seyfried F, H von Rahden B, D Miras A, Gasser M, Maeder U, Kunzmann V et al. Incidence, time course and independent risk factors for metachronous peritoneal carcinomatosis of gastric origin-a longitudinal experience from a prospectively collected database of 1108 patients. *BMC Cancer* 2015;15:73.

[6] Lim B, Kim C, Kim JH, Kwon WS, Lee WS, Kim JM, Park JY, Kim HS, Park KH, Kim TS, Park JL, Chung HC, Rha SY, Kim SY. Genetic alterations and their clinical implications in gastric cancer peritoneal carcinomatosis revealed by whole-exome sequencing of malignant ascites. *Oncotarget.* 2016 Feb 16;7(7):8055-66. doi: 10.18632/oncotarget.6977. PMID: 26811494; PMCID: PMC4884975.

[7] Jayne D. Molecular biology of peritoneal carcinomatosis. *Cancer Treat. Res.* 2007; 134:21–33.

[8] Kusamura S, Baratti D, Zaffaroni N, Villa R, Laterza B, Balestra MR, Deraco M. Pathophysiology and biology of peritoneal carcinomatosis. *World J. Gastrointest. Oncol*. 2010; 2:12–18.

[9] Sangisetty SL, Miner TJ. Malignant ascites: A review of prognostic factors, pathophysiology and therapeutic measures. *World J. Gastrointest. Surg.* 2012; 4:87–95.

[10] Kuroda A, Tsukamoto Y, Nguyen LT, Noguchi T, Takeuchi I, Uchida M, Uchida T, Hijiya N, Nakada C, Okimoto T, Kodama M, Murakami K, Matsuura K, et al. Genomic profiling of submucosal-invasive gastric cancer by array based comparative genomic hybridization. *PLoS One.* 2011; 6:e22313.

[11] Cristescu, R; Lee, J; Nebozhyn, M; Kim, K M; Ting, J C; Wong, S S; Liu, J; Yue, Y G; Wang, J; Yu, K; et al. Molecular analysis of gastric

cancer identifies subtypes associated with distinct clinical outcomes. *Nat. Med.* 2015, 21, 449–456.

[12] Miao, Z F; Wang, Z N; Zhao, T T; Xu, Y Y; Gao, J; Miao, F; Xu, H M. Peritoneal milky spots serve as a hypoxic niche and favor gastric cancer stem/progenitor cell peritoneal dissemination through hipoxia-inducible factor 1α. *Stem Cells* 2014, 32, 3062–3074.

[13] D'Angelica M, Gonen M, Brennan MF, Turnbull AD, Bains M, Karpeh MS. Patterns of initial recurrence in completely resected gastric adenocarcinoma. *Ann. Surg.* 2004;240:808–816. doi: 10.1097/01.sla.0000143245.28656.15.

[14] Merchant SJ, Kim J, Choi AH, Sun V, Chao J, Nelson R. A rising trend in the incidence of advanced gastric cancer in young Hispanic men. *Gastric Cancer.* 2017;20:226–234. doi: 10.1007/s10120-016-0603-7.

[15] Valle M, Federici O, Garofalo A. Patient selection for cytoreductive surgery and hyperthermicintrapcritoneal chemotherapy, and role of laparoscopy in diagnosis, staging and treatment. *Surg. Oncol. Clin. N. Am.* 2012;21(4):515–31.

[16] Leake, Pierre-Anthony et al. A systemic review of the accuracy and indications for diagnostic laparoscopy prior to curative-intent resection of gastric cancer, *Gastric Cancer,*Febrero, 2011.

[17] Martin-Richard, M A Custodio, C Garcıa-Girón, C Grávalos, C Gomez, P Jimenez- Fonseca, J L Manzano, C Pericay, F Rivera, A Carrato. Seom guidelines for the treatment of gastric cancer 2015. *Clin. Transl. Oncol.* 2015; 17:996–1004.

[18] Smyth, E C M,Verheij, W. Allum, D. Cunningham, A. Cervantes & D. Arnold on behalf of the ESMO Guidelines Committee et al. Gastric cancer: ESMO Clinical Practice Guidelines for diagnosis, treatment and follow-up. *Ann. Oncol.* 2016; 27 (Supplement 5): v38–v49.

[19] Chua YJ, Cunningham D. The UK NCRI MAGIC trial of perioperative chemotherapy in resectable gastric cancer: implications for clinical practice. *Ann. Surg. Oncol.* 2007;14:2687-90.

[20] Roeland E, Kanter K, Wo JY-L, Fish M, Nipp RD Seventer EEV, et al. Preliminary analysis of total neoadjuvant therapy for patients with locally advanced gastric (G) and gastroesophageal (GE) adenocarcinoma. *Journal Clinical Oncology* 2020;38 (4_suppl):393.

[21] Van der Speeten K, Stuart OA, Sugarbaker PH. Pharmacology of perioperative intraperitoneal and intravenous chemotherapy in patients with peritoneal surface malignancy. *Surg. Oncol. Clin. N. Am.* 2012; 21: 577-597].

[22] Bonnot PE, Piessen G, Kepenekian V, Decullier E, Pocard M, Meunier B, Bereder JM, Abboud K, Marchal F, Quenet F, Goere D, Msika S, Arvieux C, Pirro N, Wernert R, Rat P, Gagnière J, Lefevre JH, Courvoisier T, Kianmanesh R, Vaudoyer D, Rivoire M, Meeus P, Passot G, Glehen O; FREGAT and BIG-RENAPE Networks. Cytoreductive Surgery With or Without Hyperthermic Intraperitoneal Chemotherapy for Gastric Cancer with Peritoneal Metastases (CYTO-CHIP study): A Propensity Score Analysis. *J. Clin. Oncol.* 2019 Aug 10;37(23):2028-2040. doi: 10.1200/JCO.18.01688. Epub 2019 May 14. PMID: 31084544.

[23] Bruna Esteban M, Vorwald P, Ortega Lucea S, Ramírez Rodríguez JM; Grupo de Trabajo de Cirugía Esofagogástrica del Grupo Español de Rehabilitación Multimodal (GERM). Enhanced recovery after surgery in gastric resections. *Cir. Esp.* 2017 Feb;95(2):73-82. English, Spanish. doi: 10.1016/j.ciresp.2016.10.013. Epub 2017 Feb 6. PMID: 28185641.

[24] Gemmill EH, Humes DJ, Catton JA. Systematic review of enhanced recovery after gastro-oesophageal cancer surgery. *Ann. R. Coll. Surg. Engl.* 2015;97:173–9.

[25] Siddharthan R et al. Feasibility and benefits of an enhanced recovery after surgery protocol for patients undergoing cytoreductive surgery and heated intraperitoneal chemotharpy: A single institution experience, *The American Journal of Surgery*, https:// doi.org/10.1016/j.amjsurg.2019.06.019.

[26] Yonemura Y, de Aretxabala X, Fujimura T, Fushida S, Katayama K, Bandou E, et al. Intraoperative chemohyperthermic peritoneal

perfusion as an adjuvant to gastric cancer: final results of a randomized controlled study. *Hepatogastroenterology.* 2001;48:1776–82.

[27] Kim JY, Bae HS. A controlled clinical study of serosa-invasive gastric carcinoma patients who underwent surgery plus intraperitoneal hyperthermo-chemo-perfusion (IHCP). *Gastric Cancer.* 2001;4(1):27–33.

[28] Brenkman HJF, Päeva M, van Hillegersberg R, Ruurda JP, Haj Mohammad H. Prophylactic Hyperthermic Intraperitoneal Chemotherapy (HIPEC) for Gastric Cancer—A Systematic Review. *J. Clin. Med.* 2019;8:1685.

[29] Glehen, O, Passot, G, Villeneuve, L. et al. GASTRICHIP: D2 resection and hyperthermic intraperitoneal chemotherapy in locally advanced gastric carcinoma: a randomized and multicenter phase III study. *BMC Cancer* 14, 183 (2014).

In: Gastric Peritoneal Carcinomatosis ISBN: 978-1-53619-487-6
Editors: F. López Mozos et al.

Chapter 2

ROLE OF IMAGING IN PERITONEAL SURFACE MALIGNANCIES

Almudena Vera*, MD, Ana Alcolado, MD and Sergio Torondel, MD
Department of Radiology,
Hospital Clínico Universitario, Valencia, Spain

ABSTRACT

Gastric cancer is still diagnosed at an advanced stage. The presence of peritoneal metastases has implications in the choice of treatment and prognosis. Although exploratory laparoscopy is the gold standard in the evaluation of peritoneal disease, it is an invasive procedure. Therefore, images play a vital role in the staging of peritoneal disease.

Multidetector Computed Tomography (MDCT) is widely available, fast to perform, and offers good resolution. In fact, it is the main imaging modality for complete preoperative clinical staging. Furthermore, CT is included in clinical practice guidelines for its ability to detect local or distant lymph nodes, metastasis, or peritoneal carcinomatosis.

The TNM should be applied according to the 8th latest edition of the AJCC. We describe the radiological criteria established to classify

* Corresponding Author's E-mail: almuverag@gmail.com.

patients in a specific stage to carry out the most appropriate treatment strategy.

MDCT also allows to establish the distribution, extent and preoperative estimation of the peritoneal carcinomatosis index (PCI). PCI is the prognostic score of choice for patients with advanced tumors who undergo cytoreductive surgery and hyperthermic intraperitoneal chemotherapy.

In this chapter we also review the implementation of additional imaging tools as MRI (Magnetic Resonance Imaging). Although its availability is limited and study time is longer, the development of high-speed sequences, combined morphological sequences with gadolinium-enhanced and DWI images have made MRI a feasible tool for the staging of gastric cancer and the detection of peritoneal disease.

The utility of PET remains controversial. However, we review its advantages and limitations. Due to the lower resolution of PET, small peritoneal nodules may be missed. Mucinous carcinomas, signet ring cells, and poorly differentiated adenocarcinomas have lower FDG uptake, so peritoneal metastases from these tumours could also be underdiagnosed.

Computed Tomography (CT) and TNM

Accurate staging is essential to choose the most appropriate treatment course for any patient. The tumor-node-metastasis (TNM) staging system of the 8th edition of the AJCC has been shown to accurately predict prognosis for gastric cancer patients [1].

CT and endoscopic ultrasonography (EUS) are the main imaging modalities used for the preoperative staging of gastric cancer. Multidetector CT has become the most important diagnostic tool for staging due to its ability to detect distant metastases (M) and lymph node involvement (N).

CT Protocol

CT scan is acquired in supine position, with an adequate luminal distension, using multiphasic contrast-enhanced imaging, thin-section collimation and high-quality multiplanar reformatted images.

Adequate gastric distension is mandatory and can be obtained through the use of endoluminal contrast agents. Such contrast can be of high density (positive) (diatrizoate of meglumine water solutions) or low density (negative agents) (water, air or CO_2) [2].

For CT-mediated staging of gastric cancer, water represents a simple agent with low costs and complication rates, well tolerated by patients and capable of accurately distending the gastric cavity for optimal visualization of the intestinal wall, serosa, and peritoneum [2]. Typically patients ingest 800 mL of water before CT scanning [3].

The use of a positive oral contrast may hinder the visualization of calcified serosal nodules or peritoneal tumor deposits [4].

In addition to oral contrast medium, the use of intravenous contrast is fundamental for a proper evaluation. We generally administer 100-150 ml (1.5 ml / kg of body weight) of non-ionic contrast material at a rate of 3-4 ml / sec. Then a double-phase imaging is routinely performed. Arterial phase (25 to 40 seconds after injection of intravenous contrast medium) and venous phase (at 60 to 80 seconds). Arterial phase imaging improves tumor detection, and venous phase imaging is useful for evaluating lymph nodes and distant metastases [2, 3]. To further aid in diagnosis, axial and multiplanar (coronal and sagittal) reconstructions images are examined.

Gastric carcinoma usually appears as an irregular thickening of the gastric wall and exhibits high density compared to contiguous normal walls [2]. Other suspicious findings on CT include obliteration of normal layers of the gastric wall, perigastric fat stranding, and the presence of perigastric lymph nodes [3]. Voluminous lesions may appear inhomogeneous when necrotic areas are present [2].

The degree of enhancement depends on the histological subtype and stage of the tumor, thus, mucinous tumor subtypes demonstrate relative hypoattenuation due to the presence of mucin. Signet ring cell carcinoma, a subset of diffuse-type gastric adenocarcinoma [8], presents as an infiltrative thickening leading to a scirrhous infiltration of the gastric wall (linitis plastica) [3].

TUMOR STAGING

Tumor stages are defined according to the American Joint Committee on Cancer (AJCC) 8th edition [1]. Relevant imaging reviews in the 8th edition of the AJCC Cancer Staging Manual include the classification of gastric versus esophageal cancers based on tumor location and regional versus metastatic node disease assignment.

The prognosis is associated with the anatomical location of the tumor in the stomach. If the epicenter of the tumor is located 2 cm or less below the esophagogastric junction (EGJ) it should be classified according to the esophageal cancer system (Siewert type II tumours).

The degree of wall invasion is represented by the T (tumor). The CT criteria used for the different T categories are:

- *T1:* tumor invades lamina propria, muscularis mucosae or submucosa. T1 tumors at times lack evident radiologic findings on CT. Sometimes, a focal thickening of the gastric wall with or without enhancement of the inner surface, associated to a preserved outer surface of the stomach can be demonstrated. A significant focal enhancement in the gastric wall without thickening can also be a sign of a T1 tumor.
- *T2:* tumor invades muscularis propria. The entire gastric wall where the lesion is located will be fully enhanced and will display significant thickening, whilst maintaining a clear external border with the regional fat. (Figure 1)
- *T3:* tumor penetrates the subserosal connective tissue without invasion of the visceral peritoneum or adjacent structures: the serosal contour becomes blurred, and stranded areas of greater attenuation may be seen extending into the perigastric fat [2]. (Figure 2)
- *T4:* tumor invades the serosa (visceral peritoneum) or adjacent structures. Tumor spread frequently occurs via ligamentous and peritoneal reflections to adjacent organs. The transverse colon may

be affected through the gastrocolic ligament, pancreas by the lesser sac and the liver along the gastrohepatic ligament [2]. (Figure 3)

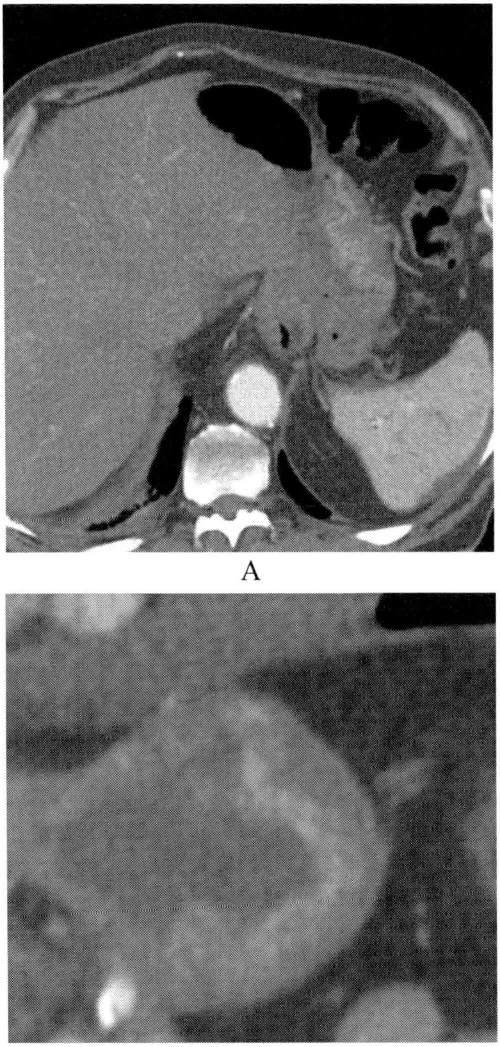

A

B

Figure 1. T2N0. A) Axial contrast-enhanced CT image. Eccentric enhancement and thickening wall of greater curvature of the stomach. B) Coronal contrast-enhanced CT image. Eccentric enhancement and thickening wall with clear external border with regional fat.

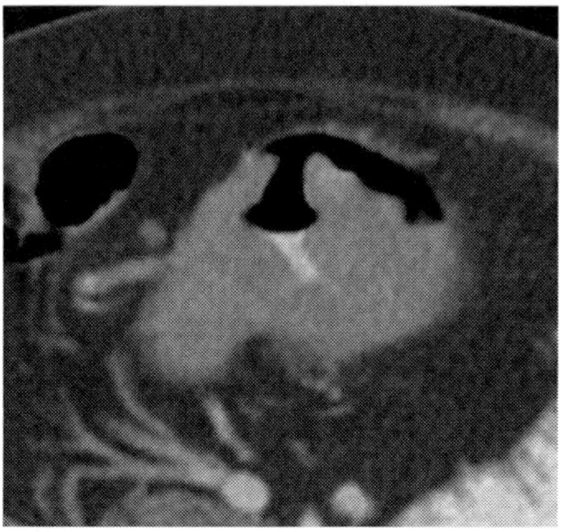

A

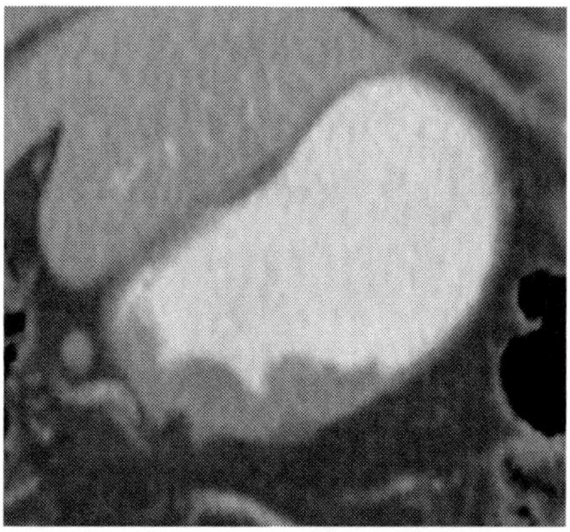

B

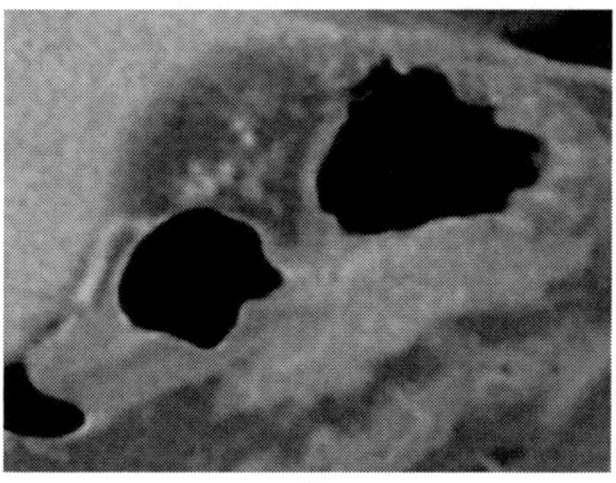

C

Figure 2. A) and B) T3.N1. Axial and Coronal contrast-enhanced CT image showing circumferential wall thickening of the gastric antrum. The serosal contour is blurred and there are areas of increased attenuation into the perigastric fat. C) T3. Coronal image. Wall thickening of the greater curvature with extension into the perigastric fat.

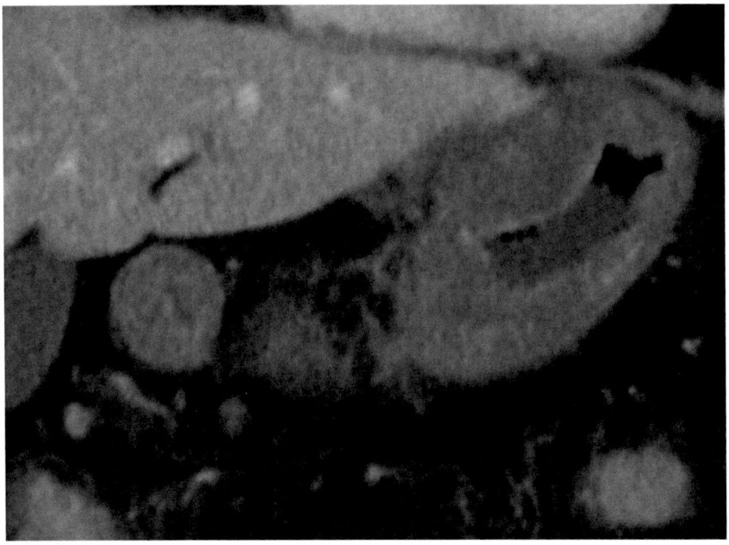

Figure 3. T4. Coronal contrast-enhanced CT image. Tumor invades the liver and the gastrohepatic ligament. There are two perigatric metastatic nodes in the greater curvature.

A gastric mass abutting adjacent organs and the absence of fatty plane between the mass and the organ are indicative, but not diagnostic, of organ invasion [2].

Node Staging (N)

The AJCC (American Joint Committee on Cancer) staging system establishes that a minimum of 15 nodes should be examined for correct lymph node staging [1]. Only regional lymph nodes are evaluated (Figure 4).

N staging is based on the number of positive nodes (N1, metastasis in one to two regional lymph nodes; N2, metastasis in three to six lymph nodes; and N3, metastasis in more than seven lymph nodes) N3a: Metastasis in seven to 15 regional lymph nodes and N3b: Metastasis in 16 or more regional lymph nodes.

Involvement of lymph node groups different than regional ones is considered distant metastasis (M1). Therefore, supraclavicular lymph node involvement is considered distant metastasis rather than nodal metastasis and excludes curative surgery.

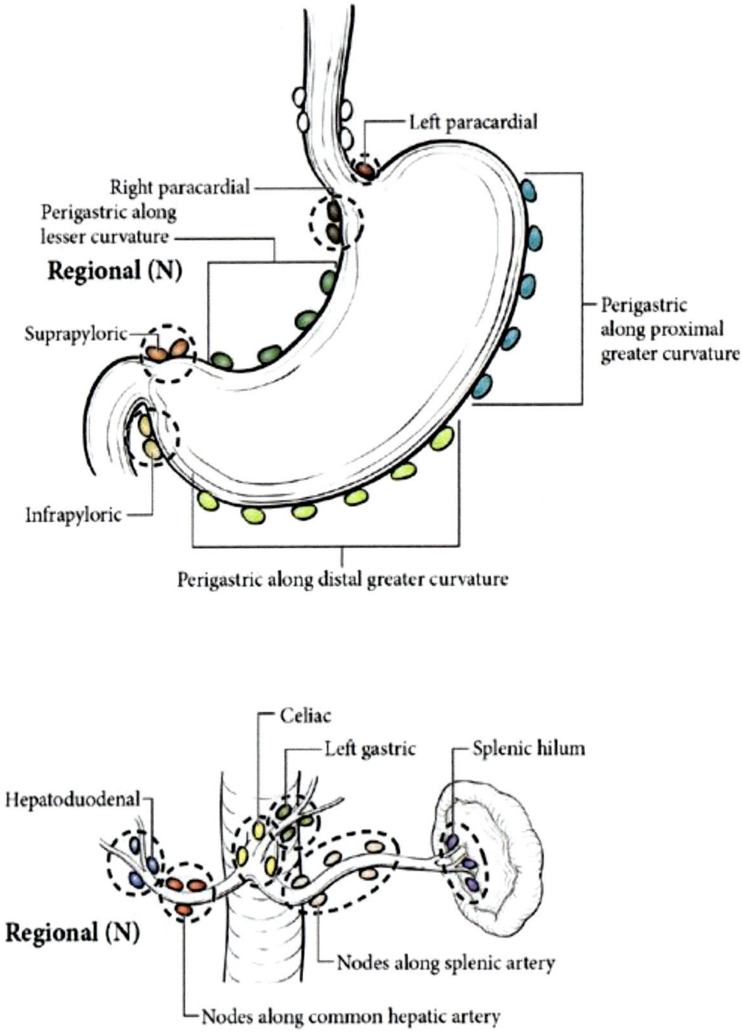

Figure 4. Regional lymph nodes of the stomach. [1]AJCC Cancer Staging Manual, Eighth Edition. 2018.

The criteria used to radiologically asses and determine the affected nodes are [2]:

- Size: more than 8-10 mm in transverse diameter. We used 8 mm of transverse diameter for perigastric location and 10 mm for the rest.
- Rounded morphology.
- Central necrosis.
- Marked or heterogeneous contrast enhancement.

The presence of these criteria specially when combined, has a strong correlation with the existence of lymph node metastases. CT has an important limitation, it cannot help detect cancerous involvement of normal-sized nodes or distinguish between reactive hyperplasia and metastatic enlargement [2].

Fluorine-18 fluoro-2-deoxy-d-glucose positron emission tomography/ computed tomography (18F-FDG PET/CT) has the ability to show changes in metabolism and could be used to overcome this limitation of CT. In addition, PET-CT can detect metastases in the extra-abdominal lymph nodes by also allowing images of the whole body [2].

Currently, endoscopic ultrasonography is routinely performed in the diagnosis of gastric cancer since it provides a very precise evaluation of the degree of parietal invasion, has the ability to differentiate T1 from T2, with a sensitivity of 85% and a specificity of 90%. Similar accuracy has been reported in differentiating a superficial tumor from an advanced tumor [13]. Nevertheless, endoscopic US also provides very good data from the evaluation of local lymph nodes and serves as a guide to puncture these suspicious nodes, increasing its sensitivity in the diagnosis up to 100% [13].

Distant Metastasis (M)

This can be M0 (no distant metastases) or M1 (distant metastases). Distant metastases (M1 disease) includes distant nodal metastases, peritoneal carcinomatosis, visceral metastases, and lymphangitic spread to the lungs.

Hematogenous metastases from gastric carcinoma most commonly involve the liver because the stomach is drained by the portal vein. Other less common sites of hematogenous spread include the lungs, adrenal glands, and skeleton. In the case of ovarian metastasis (Krukenberg tumor) three possible routes have been considered: peritoneal dissemination, lymphatic spread, and hematogenous spread [2, 3].

Peritoneal Carcinomatosis

The management of peritoneal carcinomatosis (PC) has evolved over the past years [4]. Also, CT has undergone important improvements [5] to aid in the detection of peritoneal metastases. Currently, radiologists play a fundamental role in the decision of the therapeutic strategy because they can identify patients that will be treated by means of palliative surgery or curative resection.

Up to 50% of patients with tumors penetrating the muscular layer or beyond are known to have peritoneal disease at the time of presentation [6]. In addition, up to 53% of patients who present a recurrence after curative intent resection presents in the form of peritoneal metastases [6].

Moreover, miliary PM is likely to remain undetected, even with the latest advanced CT technology. Therefore, when CT results are not definitively positive for PC, laparoscopic staging is still recommended if a patient is considered to have a larger T-stage tumor [7]. On the other hand, the diffuse histological type of gastric adenocarcinoma can manifest with peritoneal metastases without an easily identifiable gastric lesion. This finding leads to suspicion of a gastric origin and a gastroscopy is recommended to rule it out [6].

Although laparoscopy (SL) staging and lavage cytology is the gold standard for detecting peritoneal carcinomatosis (PC), CT is the first imaging modality in the preoperative staging of gastric cancer. This is due to its wide availability, well-established techniques and protocols, good resolution, and short acquisition times.

CT has low sensitivity, although it is very specific for detecting peritoneal disease [9]. The sensitivity and specificity published in the literature by different authors show very similar results (sensitivity: 25% - 28.3%; specificity: 78% - 98.9%) [7, 9].

Some of the common CT findings in PC are [2]:

- Ascites: is the most common finding. The location of intraperitoneal spread is influenced by gravity and by the negative subdiaphragmatic pressure caused by respiratory movements [10]. Thus, the tumor often spreads to Douglas pouch or the right paracolic gutter, or to areas where a large amount of peritoneal fluid is absorbed, such as the subdiaphragmatic surface and the omentum [6]. Therefore, it is important to carefully examine these sites.
- Nodular, plaque-shaped, or infiltrative soft tissue lesion in the peritoneal fat or peritoneal surface forming small or large masses [11].
- Parietal peritoneal thickening or enhancement
- Small bowel wall thickening or distortion
- Thickening, stranding and distortion of the mesentery [11]
- Stranding and thickening of the omentum (omental cake)
- 'Scalloping' of the liver surface due to surface/subcapsular deposits.
- Calcification, if found before the onset of treatment, is indicative of a mucin- producing tumor [11], [6].

We must emphasize that the size and extension of the peritoneal disease do not influence the definition of the term PC.

The use of CT in the identification of peritoneal metastases is limited by its different sensitivities, which depend on factors such as:

- The size, location, and morphological features of the tumor deposit [2]:
- Tumor deposits of less than 5 mm, those located in the root of the mesentery, lesser omentum, left hemidiaphragm and the serous surface of the bowel have a low sensitivity to be detected by CT scan (11–48%) [11].
- Presence of ascites
- The paucity of intra-abdominal fat
- The adequacy of bowel enhancement [2].

Peritoneal Cancer Index

The role of surgical therapy in peritoneal metastatic gastric carcinoma is still unclear. However, there is evidence that certain patients with limited peritoneal metastasis may benefit from maximal surgical therapy. The problem so far is the identification of suitable patients [12]. Therefore, imaging techniques play a decisive role in patient´s treatment planning.

From the 2000s to the present, the combination of cytoreductive surgery (CRS) with hyperthermic intraperitoneal chemotherapy (HIPEC) has been gaining popularity, nowadays this is the standard treatment for pseudomyxoma peritonei, peritoneal mesothelioma and in selected cases of PC from colorectal cancer. Its use in PC from ovarian and gastric origin is still under investigation, but preliminary results are promising [14].

As mentioned above, CT is performed for local staging but also to measure the distant extent of the tumor. Although different imaging techniques have been used to assess preoperatively the extent and localization of peritoneal carcinomatosis (PC), a recent meta-analysis has described CT as the best imaging modality [15].

Many scores have been proposed to objectively quantify the extent of the disease. A commonly adopted score is the Peritoneal Cancer Index (PCI), first proposed by Sugarbaker to standardize the quantification of peritoneal spread. It is widely used to guide therapeutic strategies and it is correlated with the probability of complete cytoreduction and patient´s prognosis [16]. CT-PCI has a moderate but statistically significant correlation with true intraoperative PCI.

CT and surgical PCI correlation have been the object of multiple studies and metanalysis, with overestimation rates reported to range from 7% to 12% [31-32] thus recommending that CT be the image modality of choice to preoperatively asses tumor load in patients with peritoneal carcinomatosis of various origins [30].

The current description of PCI divides the abdominal cavity into 13 regions (Figure 5).

Radiologists use a standardized report template to calculate the PCI score [15]. Two components are involved in its calculation. One component is the distribution of the tumor in the abdominopelvic regions, and the other is the size of the lesion. The distribution of implants on the abdominal and pelvic surfaces influences the likelihood of complete debulking by visceral resections and peritonectomy procedures. Primary tumors or recurrences located in the surgical site, which can be excised on bloc, are excluded from the evaluation of the size of the lesion [17].

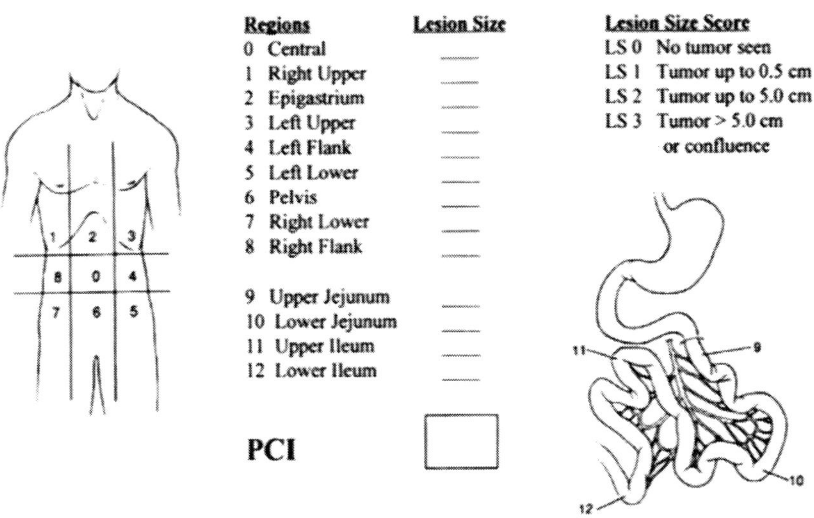

Figure 5. Sugarbaker scheme or the quantitative determination of PCI. (From Jacquet and Sugarbaker) [21].

To measure the size of the lesion, the largest diameter is employed. If there are many implants within one region, we must choose the diameter of the largest implant (17). Implants are scored as lesion size from 0 to 3 (LS-0 to LS-3):

LS-0: no implants.
LS-1: implants up to 0,5 cm.
LS-2: nodules between 0,5 to 5 cm.
LS-3: lesions greater than 5 cm. (Figure 6)

In addition, if there is confluent disease matting either abdominal or pelvic structures, it is scored as LS-3 even in present of can be interpreted as a small layer of tumor deposit [17-29].

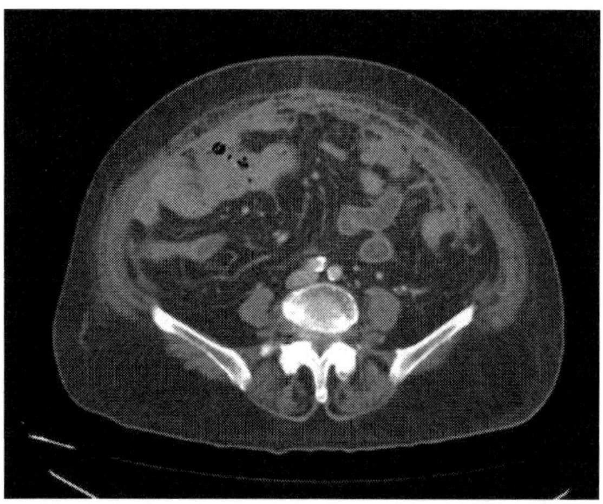

Figure 6. Omental cake with a size greater than 5 cm, LS3.

Regions 9 to 12 assess the involvement of the mesentery and small intestine, giving a score of 0 to normal appearance, a score of 1 if the small intestine and mesenteric surface are separated by fluid accumulation, and a score of 2 to the solid tumor that lines the surface of the bowel or mesentery. Segmental obstruction of the bowel is also scored as 2.

The extent of the disease can be summed as a numerical score from 0 to 39. Finally the results are compared with macroscopic and histological data after CRS and HIPEC [18], but the sensitivity of CT for malignant nodules less than 5 mm remains low, especially on surfaces of the small intestine.

The two radiological findings that Sugarbaker et al. reported as most strongly associated with a poor outcome are tumor nodules larger than 5 cm on the surface of the small intestine or directly adjacent to the bowel at the mesentery and segmental obstruction. A worse outcome has also been reported in association with extensive disease in the right upper quadrant [4].

Several recent studies have proposed a PCI of 7 as a cutoff point for selecting patients for CRS and HIPEC in peritoneal carcinomatosis from gastric origin [14].

The proximity of the tumor deposit to local structures (bowel, stomach, ureter and others) and its involvement should be carefully evaluated to indicate or not the surgery.

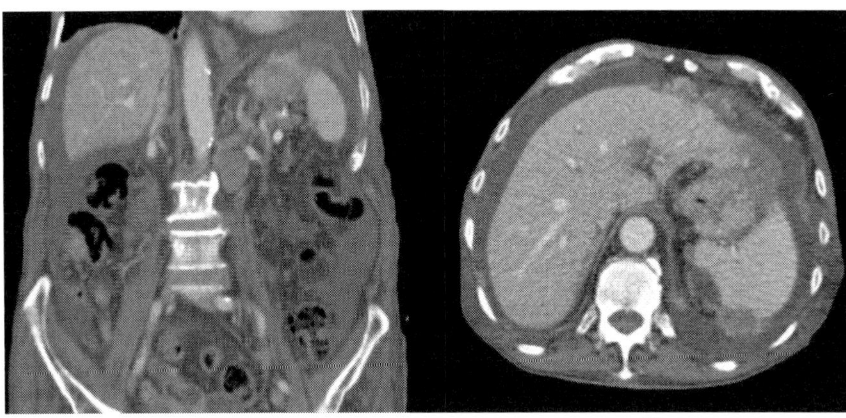

A B

Figure 7. Gastric cancer with peritoneal implants that actually invade the hepatic and splenic parenchyma, contraindicating surgery. A.- Coronal Plane. B.- Axial Plane.

For these complex cases, multimodality imaging may be required for a better planning of the therapeutic approach.

Preoperative CT has several benefits compared to MRI, including lower cost and shorter acquisition times, which makes CT easier for patients to tolerate than MRI [19].

Other Imaging Modalities

Although CT is considered the gold standard imaging technique for the study of peritoneal metastases other techniques can be considered complementary.

Magnetic Resonance Imaging (MRI) has been shown significantly better than CT in displaying contrast between different tissues, but with a lower spatial resolution.

Diffusion-weighted MRI (DWI-MRI) is a functional imaging technique based on the different mobility of protons (H +) in water. In tumor tissue, mobility tends to be limited due to increased cellularity that causes low apparent diffusion coefficients and high signal intensities in images with high b-values, in contrast to normal tissue [23](Figure 9-B).

DWI-MRI improves the detection of tumor deposits, particularly when there is mesenteric and serous involvement [23]. It is highly accurate in detecting non-operable patients, although it is less accurate in special subtypes of neoplasia, such as signet ring cells and mucinous adenocarcinoma due to its limitation to diffusion restriction. Some studies report the same accuracy in estimating PCI as laparoscopy and suggest that it could be used to select patients who are candidates for complete resection [25].

A study conducted in the Netherlands (for PC of various origins) found the correlation between DWI-MRI PCI and surgical PCI to be significantly stronger than CT estimated PCI, without patient overestimation and a sensitivity of 100% for DWI-MRI in cases with PCI lower than 21 [33]. Despite the lower availability of MRI when compared to CT, this promising results show that this technique could be a more than adequate non-invasive tool to guide selection of patients with peritoneal carcinomatosis, especially in those with borderline resectable disease.

PET-CT is an imaging technique that combines PET with a lower dose CT scan than those performed for diagnostic purposes. 18FDG (fluoro-2-deoxy-D-Glucose)) is a positron emitter that acts as a glucose analog, competing with glucose for its intracellular transport through the GLUT 1 and 3 receptors. After being phosphorylated by hexokinase, FDG phosphate cannot participate in glycolysis and remains trapped within the cell. Cells presenting a greater metabolic activity, such as neoplastic cells, will accumulate a greater amount of FDG, and this can be detected by PET-CT [28].

18FDG (fluoro-2-deoxy-D-Glucose) PET-CT has the ability to improve the detection of peritoneal metastases, especially small implants that are difficult to visualize on CT or MRI. This is due to the high metabolic activity of the lesion and the low activity of the background [23] (Figure 8).

It has greater sensitivity in the detection of peritoneal carcinomatosis than FDG-PET and CT alone and greater specificity than FDG-PET, being equal to that of CT. Numerous studies looking at the efficacy of PET, fused PET/CT (unenhanced CT) and PET/ MDCT for peritoneal malignancies imaging have yielded irregular results with sensitivity ranging from 58 to 100% [34].

A SUV (standardized uptake value) greater than 5.1 has been shown to be useful but not completely accurate in distinguishing peritoneal carcinomatosis from benign processes.

On 18 FDG PET-CT the implants appear as soft tissue nodules with increased metabolic activity, confluent nodules lining the intestine and abdominal viscera and diffuse omental peritoneal thickening (omental cake). The latter is visualized with diffuse omental thickening, nodular hyperdensity, and high and diffuse uptake of 18FDG (Figure 9-A).

In lesions with both cystic and solid component, abnormal uptake is observed in the solid part. Cystic or mucinous lesions may have low attenuation and low affinity for 18 FDG simulating loculated fluid [23, 24].

False-negative results may appear in presence of small tumor deposits, mucinous tumors (ovarian or colonic) and signet ring cell gastric cancers not taking up [18F] FDG [35]. Also cystic lesions, ascites, or miliary peritoneal involvement should be highlighted as possible causes of false negative results for this technique.

Benign peritoneal processes can have a moderate or high uptake of FDG compared to the metabolic activity of the rest of the structures or background, simulating malignant peritoneal pathology. This can occur in lymph node involvement during active inflammatory or infectious processes, in abscesses (the latter typically with a ring enhancement of FDG activity) and in post-surgical changes [23, 24].

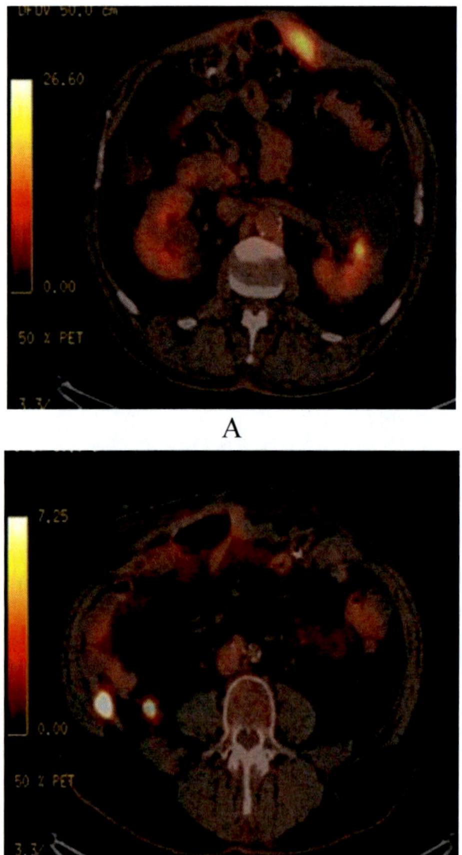

Figure 8. 18FDG PET CT study. Peritoneal implants with hypermetabolism in the anterior abdominal wall (A) and in the right lateroconal fascia (B).

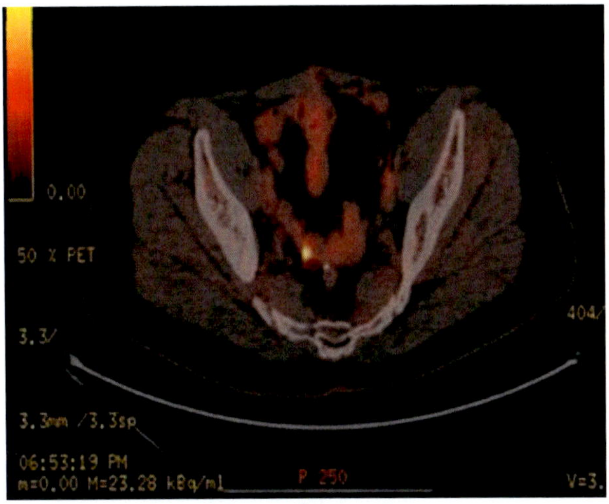

A

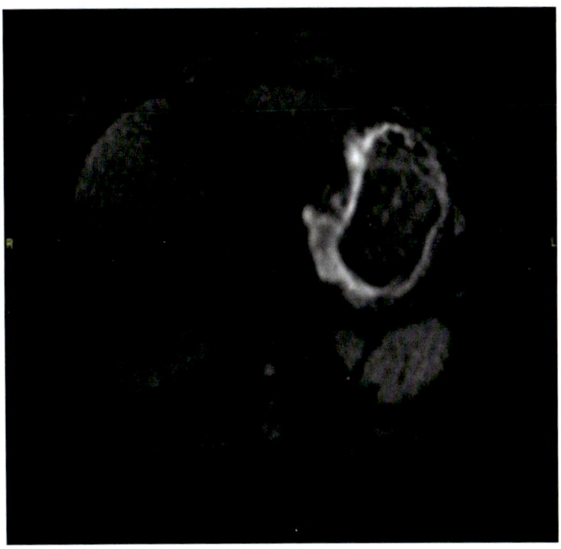

B

Figure 9. 18FDG PET CT study. A) Peritoneal implant with hypermetabolism in the small bowel loop wall. B) DWI-RM study. Restriction of gastric wall diffusion.

CONCLUSION

The management of peritoneal carcinomatosis in gastric cancer has evolved rapidly in recent years with the use of CRS and HIPEC.

Radiologists play a very important role in selecting patients for different treatment options. Currently CT has a global use, it is the best imaging technique to evaluate the local and distant extension of the tumor, using PCI as a preoperative evaluation, but other imaging modalities can be considered to improve this assessment.

REFERENCES

[1] *AJCC Cancer Staging Manual*, Eighth Edition. 2018.

[2] Joon Seok Lim, Mi Jin Yun, Myeong Jin Kim, Woo Jin Hyung, Mi-Suk Park, Jin-Young Choi, Tae-Sung Kim, Jong Doo Lee, Sung Hoon Noh, Ki Whang Kim. CT and PET in Stomach Cancer: Preoperative Staging and Monitoring of Response to Therapy. *Radio Graphics* 2006; 26:143–156.

[3] Miller F H, Kochman M L, Talamonti M S, Ghahremani G G, Gore R M. Gastric cancer. Radiologic staging. *Radiol. Clin. North Am.* 1997 Mar;35(2):331-49.

[4] Emily A. Aherne, Helen M. Fenlon Conor J. Shields, Jurgen J. Mulsow. What the Radiologist Should Know About Treatment of Peritoneal Malignancy. *American Journal of Roentgenology.* 2017;208: 531-543.

[5] Leeman M F, Patel D, Anderson J, O'Neill J R, Paterson-Brown S. Multidetector Computed Tomography Versus Staging Laparoscopy for the Detection of Peritoneal Metastases in Esophagogastric Junctional and Gastric Cancer. *Surg Laparosc Endosc Percutan Tech.* 2017 Oct;27(5):369-374.

[6] Jennifer J. Young, Anokh Pahwa, Maitraya Patel, Cecilia M. Jude, Michael Nguyen, Monica Deshmukh, Lizhou Huang, Shaden F.

Mohammad, Ligaments and Lymphatic Pathways in Gastric Adenocarcinoma. *Radio Graphics.* Vol. 39, N. 3. 2019.

[7] Su Jin Kim, Hyung-Ho Kim, Young Hoon Kim, Sun Hwi Hwang, Hye Seung Lee, Do Joong Park, So Yeon Kim, Kyoung Ho Lee. Peritoneal Metastasis: Detection with 16– or 64–Detector Row CT in Patients Undergoing Surgery for Gastric Cancer. *Radiology*: Volume 253. Number 2—November 2009.

[8] Hu B, El Hajj N, Sittler S, Lammert N, Barnes R, Meloni-Ehrig A. Gastric cancer: classification, histology and application of molecular pathology. *J. Gastrointest. Oncol.* 2012;3(3):251–261.

[9] Burbidge S, Mahady K, and Naik K. The role of CT and staging laparoscopy in the staging of gastric cancer. *Clinical radiology*, 2012. 68.

[10] Le, O. Patterns of peritoneal spread of tumor in the abdomen and pelvis. *World J. Radiol.* 2013 March 28; 5(3): 106-112.

[11] Krishnamurthy S, Balasubramaniam R. Role of Imaging in Peritoneal Surface Malignancies. *Indian J. Surg. Oncol.* (December 2016) 7(4):441–452.

[12] Hotopp T. HIPEC and CRS in peritoneal metastatic gastric cancer-who really benefits? *Surgical Oncology* 28 (2019) 159-166.

[13] Voron T, Romain B, Bergeat D. et al. Surgical management of gastric adenocarcinoma. Official expert recommendations delivered under the aegis of the French Association of Surgery (AFC). *Journal of Visceral Surgery* (2020) 157, 117-126.

[14] Manzanedo I, Pereira F, Rihuete C, et al. Surgery and Hyperthermic Intraperitoneal Chemotherapy (HIPEC) for Gastric Cancer with Peritoneal Carcinomatosis: Multicenter Study of Spanish Group of Peritoneal Oncologic Surgery (GECOP). *Ann. Surg. Oncol.* (2019) 26:2615-2621.

[15] Abdalla Ahmed S, Abou-Taleb H, Noha Ali, Dalia M. Badary. Accuracy of radiologic-laparoscopic peritoneal carcinomatosis categorization in the prediction of surgical outcome. *Br. J. Radiol.* 2019 92. 20190163.

[16] Avesani G, Arshad M, Lu H, et al. Radiological assessment of Peritoneal Cancer Index on preoperative CT in ovarian cancer is related to surgical outcome and survival. *Radiol. Med.* 2020 Aug; 125 (8):770-776.

[17] Gilly F N, Cotte E, Brigand C, Monneuse O, Beaujard AC, Freyer G, Glehen O. Quantitative prognostic indices in peritoneal carcinomatosis. *EJSO* 2006, 597-601.

[18] Mazzei M. A, Khader L, Cirigliano A, et al. Accuracy of MDCT in the preoperative definition of Peritoneal Cancer Index (PCI) in the patients with advanced ovarian cancer who underwent peritonectomy and hyperthermic intraperitoneal chemotherapy (HIPEC). *Abdom. Imaging* (2013) 38:1422-1430.

[19] Lee, R. M, Zaidi, M Y, Gamboa A C, Speegle S, Kimbrough C W, Cloyd J M, et al. What is the Optimal Preoperative Imaging Modality for Assessing Peritoneal Cancer Index? An Analysis From the United States HIPEC Collaborative. *Clinical Colorectal Cancer* 2019.

[20] Montori G, Coccolini F, Ceresoli M et al. The Treatment of Peritoneal Carcinomatosis in Advanced Gastric Cancer: State of the ART. *International Journal of Surgical Oncology*, vol 2014, Article ID 912418, 7 pages.

[21] Jacquet P, Sugarbaker P H (1996). Clinical research methodologies in diagnosis and staging of patients with peritoneal carcinomatosis. *Cancer Tr. Res.* 82.359-374.

[22] Dresen R C, De Vuysere S, De Keyzer F et al. Whole-Body diffusion Weighted MRI for operability assessment in patients with colorectal cancer and peritoneal metastases. *Cancer Imaging* (2019) 19: 1.

[23] Calderón A, Cuéllar D. PET/CT 18F-FDG en carcinomatosis peritoneal: revisión de la fisiopatología y presentación de dos casos. *Rev. Colombiana de cancerología.* 2018; 22 (2) 92-95. [18F-FDG PET / CT in peritoneal carcinomatosis: review of the pathophysiology and presentation of two cases. *Colombian Rev. of Cancerology*]

[24] Dromain C, Leboulleux S, Auperin A, et al. Stageing of peritoneal carinomatosis. Enhanced CT vs. PET/CT. *Abdominal Imaging* (2008) 33: 87-93.

[25] Engbersen M, Sant I, Lok Cet al. MRI with diffusion-weighted imaging to predict feasibility of complete cytorreduction with the peritoneal cancer index in advance stage ovarian cancer patients. *European Journal of Radiology* 114 (2019) 1: 146-151.

[26] Klumpp B D, Aschoff P, Schwenzer N et al. Peritoneal carcinomatosis: comparison of dynamic contrast-enhanced MRI with surgical and histopathologic findings. *Abdominal Imaging* (2012) 37: 834-842.

[27] Dohan A, Hoeffel C, Soyer P et al. *Evaluation of the peritoneal carcinomatosis index with CT and MRI.* 2017 BJS Society Ltd.

[28] Mandell, J. *Core Radiology. A visual approach to diagnostic imaging*. 2013. 7: 554-555.

[29] Abdalla Ahmed S, Abou-Taleb H, Ali N, M Badary D. Accuracy of radiologic- laparoscopic peritoneal carcinomatosis categorization in the prediction of surgical outcome. *Br. J. Radiol.* 2019 Aug; 92(1100):20190163.

[30] Laghi A, Bellini D, Rengo M, Accarpio F, Caruso D, Biacchi D, et al. Diagnostic performance of computed tomography and magnetic resonance imaging for detecting peritoneal metastases: systematic review and meta-analysis. *Radiol. Med.* 2017; 122: 1–15.

[31] 31 Koh J-L, Yan T D, Glenn D, Morris D L. Evaluation of preoperative computed tomography in estimating peritoneal cancer index in colorectal peritoneal carcinomatosis. *Ann. Surg. Oncol.* 2009; 16: 327–33.

[32] Esquivel J, Chua T C, Stojadinovic A, Melero J T, Levine E A, Gutman M, et al. Accuracy and clinical relevance of computed tomography scan interpretation of peritoneal cancer index in colorectal cancer peritoneal carcinomatosis: a multi-institutional study. *J. Surg. Oncol.* 2010; 102: 565–70.

[33] Van't Sant I, van Eden W J, Engbersen M P, Kok N F M, Woensdregt K, Lambregts D M J, Shanmuganathan S, Beets-Tan R

G H, Aalbers AGJ, Lahaye MJ. Diffusion-weighted MRI assessment of the peritoneal cancer index before cytoreductive surgery. *Br. J. Surg.* 2019 Mar;106(4):491-498.

[34] Patel C M, Sahdev A, Reznek R H. CT, MRI and PET imaging in peritoneal malignancy. *Cancer Imaging.* 2011 Aug 24;11(1):123-39.

[35] Anthony M P, Khong P L, Zhang J. Spectrum of (18)F-FDG PET/CT appearances in peritoneal disease. *AJR Am. J. Roentgenol.* 2009; 193: W523_9.

In: Gastric Peritoneal Carcinomatosis
Editors: F. López Mozos et al.
ISBN: 978-1-53619-487-6

Chapter 3

Diagnosis and Staging in Advanced Gastric Cancers

Benjamin L. Green and Jeremy L. Davis*
Center for Cancer Research, National Cancer Institute,
NIH, Bethesda, Maryland, US

Abstract

Gastric neoplasms comprise a diverse group of pathology with complex management choices. Accurate diagnosis and proper staging are the sine qua non of successful cancer therapy. Here we review diagnostic and staging techniques for advanced gastric tumors with an emphasis on gastric adenocarcinoma. Consideration is also given to diagnostic studies of gastrointestinal stromal tumors (GIST) and carcinoid.

* Corresponding Author's E-mail: jeremy.davis@nih.gov.

Introduction

Gastric tumors are a significant global health burden that may be minimally symptomatic well into advanced stages. Here we review the clinical, molecular, radiographic, and surgical diagnosis and staging of gastric adenocarcinoma. Gastric adenocarcinoma represents a staging conundrum; the most common site of metastatic spread is the peritoneum, frequently a radiographically occult location. This potential space can harbor tumor deposits and free cancer cells that are undetectable by current cross-sectional and nuclear imaging and would preclude a curative resection were they discovered. Diagnostic laparoscopy with peritoneal lavage has become the standard method of detecting occult peritoneal metastasis and is associated with a reduced rate of futile laparotomy for patients with stage IV disease. The molecular diagnostics and targeted therapies for gastric adenocarcinoma are less robust than those of gastric neuroendocrine tumor and gastrointestinal stromal tumor, also reviewed here. While molecular and genetic advancements hold promise to reduce the burden of disease, surgery with peri-operative chemotherapy currently represents the only curative treatment strategy for advanced non-metastatic adenocarcinoma.

Encouragingly, the global burden of gastric adenocarcinoma has been decreasing for the last 50 years [1]. This multifactorial reduction in disease incidence has been attributed to screening programs in endemic areas and better hygiene with eradication of *Helicobacter pylori* (*H. pylori*) [2]. Despite advances with biologic and targeted therapies, the median overall 5-year survival for gastric adenocarcinoma of all stages is approximately 30% in the USA, 12% in Asia, and 26% in Europe [3]. Almost no patients live 5 years past diagnosis of stage IV disease [4]. In part, this may be attributed to the observation that patients can harbor clinically silent disease for years and commonly present with advanced tumors, at least in geographic regions where screening is not employed [5].

Molecular diagnosis as an adjunct to histopathology has become increasingly important in both the diagnosis and treatment of gastric tumors. As a model of targeted therapy, the treatment of advanced gastrointestinal stromal tumor (GIST) now focuses on *KIT* gene mutation status to guide selection of tyrosine kinase inhibitor (TKI) therapy [6]. Similarly, staging and therapy for subtypes of gastric neuroendocrine tumors (GNET) take advantage of the unique affinity of somatostatin for neuroendocrine tumor cells [7]. Treatments for individual gastric adenocarcinoma molecular subtypes, meanwhile, are less well-defined. Biologic and targeted therapies have been approved for treatment of advanced gastric adenocarcinoma, such as inhibition of human epidermal growth factor receptor 2 (HER2) [8], vascular endothelial growth factor receptor 2 (VEGFR2) [9], and programmed death-ligand 1 (PD-L1) [10]. Both new and existing therapies rely upon accurate diagnosis and staging of gastric adenocarcinoma.

Clinical Presentation and Diagnosis

Symptoms

The majority of patients with early stage disease are asymptomatic whereas clinical symptoms of gastric cancer frequently occur at later stages [11, 12]. As tumor stage advances, patients can present with subtle abdominal symptoms often indistinguishable from benign pathology such as dyspepsia, gastroesophageal reflux, or epigastric pain [13]. Symptoms concerning for advanced disease are anorexia, unintentional weight loss, early satiety, and vomiting [14]. The number of alarm symptoms on presentation has been found to correlate with stage and survival [15]. Any ongoing dyspepsia in patients that are refractory to antiulcer medications and/or those over a certain age is suspicious [16]. The exact age to use as a cutoff to refer for endoscopy is variable, with a lower age threshold used in certain endemic areas of Asia (i.e., less than 45 years old) [17]. A detailed family history should be performed, and any gastric adenocarcinoma in first- or second-degree relatives further raises suspicion. In the USA specifically, Latin American [18] and Alaskan Native [19] populations have a higher risk of gastric cancer as compared to other populations.

Certain symptoms correlate with tumor location. For instance, dysphagia is more characteristic of gastroesophageal junction (GEJ) tumors, while gastric outlet obstruction occurs more often with antral tumors. Both alarm symptoms in normal-risk patients and non-specific symptoms in high-risk patients should trigger expeditious workup including endoscopy.

Signs

Physical exam is non-specific for diagnosis of gastric adenocarcinoma. Chronic and major weight loss may be observed, which can appear with muscle wasting and cachexia. Signs of malignant bowel obstruction, such as abdominal distention and palpable abdominal mass, fluid wave from ascites, and melena due to gastrointestinal (GI) blood loss can be part of acute clinical presentation of advanced gastric cancer. Classic exam findings of advanced abdominal malignancy may be uncommon. Lymphadenopathy at Virchow's node is due to metastasis through the thoracic duct to a supraclavicular station [20]; Sister Mary Joseph's nodule is a visible umbilical metastasis from direct peritoneal spread. Both eponymous signs occur in a minority of patients and are generally markers of advanced disease [21]. Drop metastasis can be appreciated in Blumer's shelf, a mass palpable on digital rectal exam in the rectouterine or rectovesical pouch, though this sign is also uncommon.

Laboratory Studies

Laboratory abnormalities are a frequent corroborating finding in patients presenting with gastric adenocarcinoma. Iron-deficiency anemia can originate from occult upper GI bleeding [22]. Other findings of chronic malnutrition include a decrease in serum albumin and elevated international normalized ratio. Gastric outlet obstruction (GOO) can present acutely with electrolyte abnormalities including hypochloremic metabolic alkalosis, as well as acute kidney injury. Electrolyte and nutritional abnormalities should be corrected. In patients with GOO, a feeding jejunostomy tube and/or decompressive gastrostomy tube can be effective in relieving symptoms, improving nutritional status, and optimizing patients for subsequent chemotherapy or surgery [23].

Analysis of serum tumor markers is not recommended by the National Comprehensive Cancer Network (NCCN) guidelines for gastric adenocarcinoma, as rates of elevation are inconsistent for patients with early stage disease. In one meta-analysis, carcinoembryonic antigen (CEA), carbohydrate antigen 19-9 (CA19-9), and carbohydrate antigen 72-4 (CA72-4) were elevated in only 21-30% of patients with gastric adenocarcinoma [24]. However, tumor markers appear to be elevated in late stage disease [25] and they may have prognostic value. When elevated at diagnosis, CA19-9 and CEA have a negative association with survival. Postoperatively, elevated CEA and CA19-9 levels were found to be independent negative prognostic factors for overall survival [26]. In one study, CEA that normalized following surgery did not correlate with improved overall survival, yet normalized postoperative CA19-9 levels correlated with better overall survival [27]. As described later, CEA mRNA is being evaluated for its sensitivity to detect occult tumor cells in peritoneal lavage specimens.

Endoscopy

Upper endoscopy with biopsy is the gold standard for obtaining the diagnosis of gastric adenocarcinoma and should be recommended in all patients suspected for gastric malignancy [28]. The entire mucosa of the esophagus, the stomach, and at least the first two portions of the duodenum should be examined presuming obstruction is absent (Figure 1A). Any suspicious lesions, ulcers, or polyps should be biopsied using cold forceps or snare as appropriate. A total of 6-8 tissue samples from the viable borders of any ulcer should be obtained as this range is 98% sensitive for detection of malignancy [29]. Tissue procured during an endoscopy should be labeled separately, fixed, and analyzed for neoplastic features and well as *H. pylori* infection. The diagnostic accuracy of endoscopy for early gastric adenocarcinoma is over 90% [30]. Endoscopic appearance of lesions can be indicative of their malignancy potential. More often, benign gastric ulcers have a symmetric appearance, even bases, sharply demarcated borders, and rugal folds running perpendicular to the tangent of the ulcer. Malignant ulcers appear irregular, asymmetric, thick-bordered, or necrotic. Hemorrhagic gastric neoplasms can present as a mass or ulcer. Patients with an upper GI bleed should undergo endoscopy for hemostasis. Biopsies of suspicious tissue can then be obtained concurrently or via repeat procedure depending on hemodynamic stability.

The Paris and Borrmann classification systems are used to describe morphology of endoscopically discovered early and advanced lesions, respectively. Early lesions are described as Paris type 0-I for polypoid (pedunculated or sessile), 0-II for superficial (elevated, flat, or depressed), and 0-III for excavated [31]. Advanced lesions are described as Borrmann type I (polypoid), type II (fungating), type III (ulcerated), or type IV (infiltrative). Borrmann type IV, often located near the antrum, carries a particularly poor prognosis, as its mucosal and submucosal spread indicates an aggressive biology [32].

Linitis plastica, often confused for but not mutually exclusive with Borrmann type IV, is a scirrhous phenotype of advanced-stage adenocarcinoma with a characteristic longitudinal spread along the muscularis propria layer, with or without mucosal involvement. Endoscopic appearance of linitis plastica is thickening of the gastric wall, with poor distensibility on insufflation and stiffening of at least one-third of the stomach (Figure 1B) [33]. Intramural spread makes the diagnosis of linitis plastica challenging. Grossly and microscopically normal mucosa on endoscopy and biopsy can mask adenocarcinoma cells in the muscularis layer, causing variable accuracy of mucosal biopsy in detecting linitis plastica. Stiff insufflation, "cobblestone" mucosal surface, or hypertrophy of the mucosal folds are endoscopic features that should be concerning when present. Advanced biopsy techniques such as tunnel biopsies, snare, endoscopic ultrasound (EUS)-guided core biopsies, or mucosal resections can reveal malignant cells within the stomach wall, and should be performed when suspicion is high [28]. As with Borrmann type IV, linitis plastica carries a poor prognosis due to aggressive tumor biology [33].

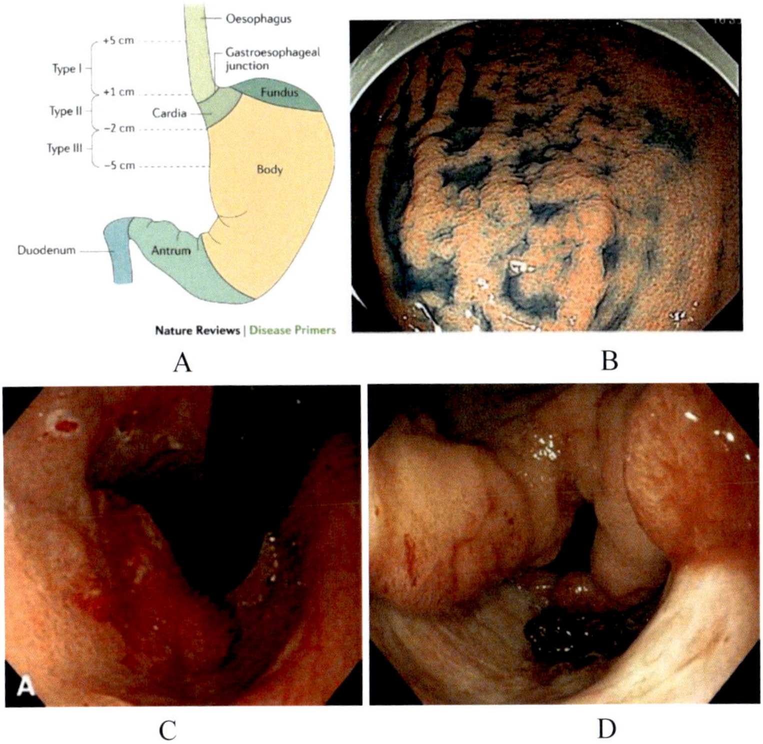

Figure 1. Anatomic and endoscopic characteristics of gastric adenocarcinoma. A. Schematic of Siewert-Stein classification, anatomic regions of stomach [1]. b. Characteristic appearance of linitis plastica [2]. c. Cardia tumor [3]. d. Antral tumor [4].

Endoscopy is also used as a surveillance technique for patients with Heredity Diffuse Gastric Cancer (HDGC), a germline mutation that increases likelihood of developing gastric adenocarcinoma, most commonly in the *CDH1* gene (see below). Biopsies of both suspicious and grossly normal mucosa are taken methodically in a topographical fashion ("gastric mapping") [34]. After obtaining biopsies from grossly abnormal tissue, five random biopsies should be taken from normal-appearing tissue in each of 6 regions of the stomach: prepyloric, antrum, transitional zone, body, fundus, and cardia. Duration of gastroscopy is at least 30 minutes with repeated insufflation to evaluate for distensibility, a potential sign of infiltrative cancer [35]. Surveillance of other hereditary gastric adenocarcinoma syndromes utilizes a similar endoscopic technique, including Gastric Adenocarcinoma and Proximal Polyposis of the Stomach (GAPPS) and Familial Intestinal Gastric Cancer (FIGC).

Diagnosis of Gastric Adenocarcinoma

Location and histology of gastric adenocarcinoma define its biology and have implications on diagnosis and management. Distal adenocarcinomas, often of intestinal-type histology, account for much of the decreasing overall incidence of gastric cancer. Proximal gastric cancers, especially those of the cardia and gastroesophageal junction (Siewert-Stein classification type III) [36] are often considered to exhibit more aggressive behavior and are increasing in incidence [37] (Figure 1C).

Histopathology

Gastric adenocarcinoma exhibits two histological phenotypes described by Laurén [38]. Intestinal type adenocarcinoma is often associated with distal tumor location. It is characterized by microscopic gland formation comparable to other GI tract adenocarcinomas. The mechanism of intestinal type neoplasia is well-described by Correa's cascade [39]. Briefly, chronic inflammation of the body or antrum induces a progression from precursor non-atrophic gastritis to atrophic gastritis, then transformation to intestinal metaplasia, dysplasia, and cancer. *H. pylori* is detectible on endoscopic biopsies using immunohistochemistry (IHC), but also via Giemsa or Warthin-Starry stains [40].

In contrast to intestinal type histology, diffuse type adenocarcinoma is associated with proximal tumor location and displays more aggressive features [41]. Microscopically, cells displaying diffuse type histology appear poorly cohesive and lack the gland formation typical of intestinal type. A subset of diffuse type histology is signet ring cells that contain large cytoplasmic mucin stores [42]. These cells can be identified through the use of periodic acid-Schiff (PAS) histochemical staining. Patients bearing pathogenic germline *CDH1* gene variants commonly have occult signet ring cell carcinomas present in the mucosa found on gastric endoscopy [43]. The presence of signet ring cells is pathognomonic of the hereditary diffuse gastric cancer syndrome due to *CDH1* gene mutation. These patients carry a 25-42% lifetime risk of advanced gastric cancer [44, 45].

Molecular Diagnosis

Molecular subclassifications of gastric adenocarcinoma have been developed based on large-scale genomic analysis. A prime example was developed by The Cancer Genome Atlas (TCGA) research network which generated four unique molecular categories of gastric adenocarcinoma: Epstein–Barr virus (EBV) positive, microsatellite-instability (MSI) high, genomically stable (GS), and chromosomal instability (CIN) [46]. These categories have helped delineate subpopulations of patients whose tumors likely arise due to different mechanisms and therefore may be susceptible to biologic or targeted therapies. Notably, there are other large-scale analyses that yielded slightly different but similarly impactful molecular subclassifications [47].

EBV-Positive and MSI High

Epstein-Barr virus can be detected using an *in situ* hybridization assay for Epstein-Barr encoding region (EBER). EBV-positive gastric tumors tend to be associated with fundus or corpus (body) tumor location. A key molecular characteristic seen in EBV-positive cancer cells is global CpG island methylation in the promoter region of many cancer-related genes. Histologically, EBV-positive gastric adenocarcinoma appears to have prominent lymphocytic infiltration [48]. For MSI high tumors, downregulation of the expression of multiple genes (e.g., *MLH1, MSH2*) involved in mismatch repair (MMR) can lead to signature microsatellite repeats throughout the genome and is associated with tumorigenesis. The diagnosis of MSI-tumor is made based on PCR detection of increased microsatellites, as well as decreased expression of MMR genes by IHC. Like EBV-positive tumors, MSI-high tumors display CpG-island hypermethylation [49].

GS and CIN

In the TCGA study, tumors lacking EBV infection and MSI were analyzed for somatic copy-number aberrations. Those with high degree of aneuploidy were classified as having CIN, though there is no uniform definition for this category of gastric adenocarcinoma. It is often associated with intestinal phenotype. Most CIN tumors are found in the GEJ or cardia. This subclass has the most frequent mutations in receptor tyrosine kinase genes such as *EGFR*, *FGFR2*, *HER2*, and *MET* [46]. Finally, the GS subclass contains tumors that are negative for EBV, MSI, and CIN. Most of these tumors display the diffuse Lauren phenotype. Mutations in genes encoding cell adhesion proteins are common in GS gastric adenocarcinoma, including *CDH1* [50].

Implications for Therapy

The purpose of molecular testing is to provide rationale for systemic therapy targeting actionable mutations. EBV-positive and MSI high tumors are more likely to be responsive to checkpoint blockade immunotherapy such as pembrolizumab and nivolumab [51]. Chromosomally unstable tumors more commonly contain targetable tyrosine kinase mutations including human epidermal growth factor receptor 2 (HER2). Accordingly, the NCCN guidelines recommend molecular testing of MSI, MMR genes, *HER2*, EBV, and programmed death-ligand 1 (PD-L1) status once the diagnosis of adenocarcinoma has been established. Based on the results of phase 3 randomized controlled trials, pembrolizumab [52], bevacizumab

[53], apatinib [9], and trastuzumab [8] have all been approved for use in select gastric adenocarcinoma cases dependent on results of molecular testing. Unfortunately, no one agent has been shown to be curative for any molecular classification. Disease progression likely occurs through complex genetic escape mechanisms, as evidenced by the large degree of the genomic discordance between primary and metastatic tumors [54].

Diagnosis of Inherited Cancer Syndromes

Inherited cancer syndromes that predispose patients to development of gastric adenocarcinoma comprise 1-3% of all patients who develop gastric cancer. Heredity Diffuse Gastric Cancer (HDGC) syndrome is most commonly associated with a germline mutation in *CDH1*, a gene that encodes the E-cadherin protein (CD324), though other genes have been implicated. *CDH1* pathogenic variants are the most penetrant germline mutation associated with gastric cancer, such that 25-42% of patients bearing a pathogenic or likely pathogenic variant are predicted to develop cancer in their lifetime [44, 45]. International guidelines have been developed to outline optimal diagnosis and management of individuals with *CDH1* variants [34]. Other cancer syndromes associated with increased risk for gastric cancer development include gastric adenocarcinoma and proximal polyposis syndrome (GAPPS) [55] and familial intestinal gastric cancer (FIGC). Inherited cancer syndromes not specific for, but inclusive of, gastric adenocarcinoma include hereditary non-polyposis colorectal cancer (HPNCC), familial adenomatous polyposis (FAP), Puetz-Jeghers, juvenile polyposis, and Li-Fraumeni syndrome [56].

GIST

Gastric malignancy of non-epithelial origin is less common than adenocarcinoma. GIST is the most common soft tissue sarcoma and can arise throughout the GI tract via malignant transformation of the interstitial cells of Cajal [57]. Eighty percent of GIST are driven by a single mutation in the KIT proto-oncogene, while another 10% bear a platelet-derived growth factor receptor A (PDGFRA) mutation, and still another 10% have neither mutation (wild-type KIT and PDGFRA, “WT”). DOG1 and CD34 are additional surface markers useful for diagnosis. GIST is typically diagnosed via endoscopy. Due to the submucosal origin of GIST, standard endoscopic biopsy is not optimal for obtaining a tissue sample. Instead, endoscopic ultrasound-guided needle biopsy is the preferred diagnostic technique, either a fine-needle aspirate or core. Spindle cells can be seen on cytologic analysis. In rare cases of hemodynamic instability due to bleeding or perforation, surgical resection is both diagnostic and therapeutic.

Anatomic and pathologic staging factors have been shown to influence prognosis in patients with GIST. Tumor size greater than 5cm, mitotic rate greater than 5/50 per high-powered field, and non-gastric primary site are all negative prognostic factors [58, 59]. Tumor rupture, either spontaneous or iatrogenic, is also predictive of recurrence. Care must be taken not to violate the tumor capsule during surgical resection. In contrast to other sarcomas, the most common sites of metastasis are the liver and peritoneum, with lymphatic invasion being rare. Thus, the TNM staging system is not clinically useful in prognosticating GIST. Instead, a nomogram that incorporates the above factors is used to predict risk of recurrence following resection [58].

Tyrosine kinase inhibition has revolutionized systemic therapy for GIST. Consequently, mutational diagnosis is fundamentally important for the management of advanced GIST and can assist in TKI selection. For instance, KIT exon 9 and PDGFRA exon 18 D842V mutations are relatively resistant to imatinib therapy [60]. In addition, genotype-phenotype correlation with tumor location has been reported, as distal location of wild-type GIST is distinct from more proximal location of KIT-mutant GIST. As one of the few cancers arising from a single mutation in a cell surface growth factor receptor, the molecular characterization of GIST holds potential as a model for personalized cancer treatment. Ongoing research focuses on development of stronger TKIs, targeting alternative signaling pathways, understanding WT GIST biology, and incorporating immunotherapeutic strategies.

GNET

GNET, formerly called gastric carcinoid, is derived from malignant transformation of enterochromaffin-like (ECL) cells. Three categories of GNET exist [7]. Types 1 and 2 are thought to develop via elevated levels of gastrin, either due to chronic atrophic gastritis (type 1) or ectopic expression from a gastrinoma (type 2). Type 2 GNET can be associated with Zollinger-Ellison syndrome and seen in the context of a multiple endocrine neoplasia type 1 (MEN1) germline mutation. Both GNET types 1 and 2 typically present as multiple small, well-differentiated lesions with low rates of metastasis [61]. They can produce serotonin but rarely result in symptoms of carcinoid syndrome. In contrast, type 3 GNET is sporadic, not occurring the background of gastrinoma or atrophic gastritis. Type 3 GNET is generally a large (>1 cm) primary lesion and metastasizes to the liver more often than types 1 and 2. When functional, type 3 GNET secretes 5-hydroxy-tryptophan that can result in carcinoid syndrome including flushing, tachycardia, and diarrhea.

All patients should undergo endoscopy with biopsy. In addition to biopsy of the suspected sites of GNET, biopsy of the normal-appearing mucosa in the body, fundus, and antrum should be performed to help discern the tumor etiology. Analysis of normal gastric mucosa can assess for atrophic gastritis, intestinal metaplasia, ECL cell hyperplasia, G cell hyperplasia, and *H. pylori* status. A computed tomography (CT) abdomen/pelvis should also be performed to determine extent of disease, M stage, and synchronous enteropancreatic lesions. Serum laboratory measurements of gastrin and chromogranin A are generally elevated. The unique affinity of GNET for somatostatin offers diagnostic and staging options that are not possible in other tumors. Somatostatin scintigraphy studies such as ^{68}Ga-DOTA-TATE are very sensitive for NETs including GNET. Functional imaging is often used when there is concern for type 3

GNET to look for metastatic disease, or to detect postoperative recurrence [62]. Surgical resection is the mainstay of curative treatment for all GNET.

Clinical and Pathologic Staging of Gastric Adenocarcinoma

Clinical staging of advanced gastric adenocarcinoma can be challenging, especially as a common site for early metastasis is the peritoneum [63]. Although large disease burden can be detected on cross-sectional imaging, small tumor deposits can be radiographically occult resulting in improper staging and thus affect therapeutic decisions.

TNM Staging

The 8th edition of the American Joint Commission on Cancer (AJCC) TNM staging guidelines should be used for patients with gastric adenocarcinoma (Table 1). Increasingly granular anatomic, molecular, and regional variations in survival of subgroups of patients with gastric adenocarcinoma have challenged the prognostic accuracy of the generalized TNM system. Nomograms that incorporate tumor location have been developed to try to improve upon the current staging system [64]. Additionally, publication bias may be having an impact on TNM prognostic accuracy. For instance, some updates to the 8th edition of the AJCC guidelines were based on increased survival for Japanese subgroups of early stage adenocarcinoma, thought to be secondary to gastric cancer screening. This change may not be applicable to Western populations in which cancer is diagnosed at later stages, or Chinese populations about which survival data is relatively more scarce [65].

Tumor Stage

Endoscopic ultrasound (EUS) may be performed if no distant or nodal metastases are visualized on cross-sectional imaging, or if tumor stage is expected to be very early based on endoscopy. EUS is the most accurate diagnostic test for evaluation of tumor (T) stage as it can demonstrate depth of tumor invasion of the stomach better than CT (Figure 2). A large meta-analysis identified EUS as a sensitive modality for discriminating T1/2 lesions from T3/4, sensitivity of 0.86 and specificity of 0.90 [66]. With improvements in techniques of endoscopic mucosal resection for appropriate T1a lesions, EUS has value in evaluation of very early stage disease. This is particularly true for endemic areas with gastric cancer screening programs that encounter early stage cancer far more frequently than many Western countries.

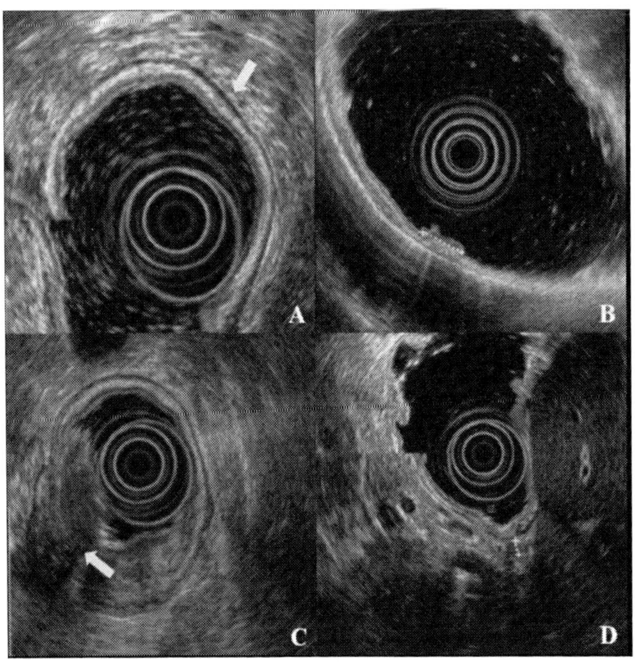

Figure 2. Endoultrasonographic images of (A) normal stomach, (B) T1a, (C) T3, and (D) Node positive gastric adenocarcinoma [5].

Table 1. AJCC 8th edition TNM staging

Category	Criteria
Tumor	
T0	No evidence of tumor
Tis	Intraepithelial tumor without invasion into lamina propria
T1a	Tumor invades into lamina propria or muscularis mucosa
T1b	Tumor invades into submucosa
T2	Tumor invades into muscularis propria
T3	Tumor invades into subserosa
T4a	Tumor invades through serosa
T4b	Tumor invades into adjacent structures
Node	
N0	No evidence of regional lymph node metastasis
N1	1-2 regional lymph node metastases
N2	3-6 regional lymph node metastases
N3a	7-15 regional lymph node metastases
N3b	16 or more regional lymph node metastases
Metastasis	
M0	No distant metastasis
M1	Distant metastasis including positive peritoneal cytology

Historically, the T stage obtained from EUS was an important determinant of the appropriateness of staging laparoscopy. Previous studies have shown improved patient selection for diagnostic laparoscopy with preoperative EUS [67]. Presently, NCCN guidelines recommend diagnostic laparoscopy to rule out peritoneal metastasis for stage greater than or equal to T1b. However, that paradigm is now being challenged in Western countries, where T stage on presentation is frequently greater than T1. Moreover, the accuracy of EUS is low for discriminating T1a from T1b, is highly user dependent, and has lower efficacy for detecting regional lymph node involvement [66]. Combined with emerging data that occult peritoneal disease is being discovered with increasing frequency in T1-2 tumors, centers are choosing to conduct other staging tests, such as laparoscopy, regardless of T stage [68].

NODE AND METASTASIS STAGING

Computed Tomography

All patients with gastric adenocarcinoma should undergo a staging CT scan to rule out metastatic disease [69]. In the setting of known metastatic disease, CT scans help quantify metastatic disease. A CT of the chest, abdomen, and pelvis with IV contrast can sensitively detect metastasis to common sites including liver, lung, and lymph nodes, and can help delineate other areas of tumor spread such as pancreas, spleen, and pelvic organs. Lymph nodes are considered clinically positive on CT if their short axis measures greater than 1 cm. For metastasis to the peritoneum, specific CT findings include omental thickening, presence of ascites, and peritoneal hyperenhancement [70]. However, the sensitivity of CT scan for peritoneal disease is low, as small deposits of tumor are often not distinguishable from adjacent soft tissue [71].

Radiomics is a rapidly developing field in which image texture is coupled with machine learning techniques to generate predictive algorithms by correlating preoperative images with postoperative pathological stage. There is significant interest in optimizing the predictive capacity of CT images to stage peritoneal metastasis non-invasively in gastric cancer. Early attempts have shown accuracy ranging from 70-90% in predicting peritoneal spread [72]. When used alone, models were inferior to the accuracy of clinic-pathologic predictions based on primary location, T stage, histology type, and differentiation [73]. However, a nomogram that combined radiomics and endoscopic features of primary tumor, peritoneum, and Lauren classification type had an accuracy of over 92% to predict peritoneal metastasis [74]. As sensitivity continues to improve, models derived from CT radiomics may be able to identify a subgroup of patients with high likelihood of advanced disease who would derive no diagnostic benefit from invasive staging procedures.

Nuclear Medicine

Fluorodeoxyglucose positron emission tomography (FDG-PET) evaluation is recommended by the NCCN for patients who do not have clear evidence of metastatic disease on CT scan. Increasingly, FDG-PET is being used for staging of lymphatic and distant organ spread. Compared with CT, FDG-PET has been shown to have superior specificity for identifying local-regional lymph node spread (92% vs. 62%) [75]. When combined, FDG-PET/CT had similar sensitivities for lymph node staging as FDG-PET alone. As discussed above, this effect may be limited to intestinal type adenocarcinoma [76]. Although FDG-PET is not sensitive for T stage, the maximum standardized uptake value (SUVmax) of an FDG-avid primary tumor may be a useful measurement for obtaining N stage. A cutoff SUVmax of 4.35 in an FDG-avid primary tumor was demonstrated to improve specificity of N stage prediction of FDG-avid lymph nodes to 92% [77]. Another study found that a primary gastric tumor SUVmax of greater than 3.2 indicated a higher likelihood of lymph node metastasis [78].

FDG-PET combined with CT is specific but not sensitive to detect occult metastatic disease. In a prospective study in which obvious metastatic disease was excluded, sensitivity of PET/CT for the detection of metastatic disease was 35%, and specificity was 99% [79]. Most frequent sites of metastatic spread identified were bone, liver, and distant lymph nodes. Importantly, FDG-PET/CT detected none of the occult peritoneal disease found by laparoscopy. Other retrospective studies have reported low sensitivity rates of FDG-PET for peritoneal metastasis [80]. Despite its ability to detect solid organ metastases, FDG-PET has low sensitivity for detecting peritoneal metastasis, necessitating further modalities for accurate staging.

FDG-PET is not meant to determine T stage. Not only does it provide limited information on histologic depth of invasion, inconsistent FDG-avidity is encountered with certain Laurén classifications of primary tumor. Intestinal type histology has higher uptake than the diffuse types, with diffuse histology and signet ring subtype displaying the lowest FDG uptake

[81]. This phenomenon is caused by reduced levels of GLUT1 transmembrane glucose transporter in diffuse type cancer cells [82]. In one series, only 44% of diffuse type were FDG-avid, while 97% of intestinal type were FDG-avid [79]. Potential PET avidity can be predicted based on a scoring system that includes size, non-signet ring cell histology, and GLUT1 expression as measured by immunohistochemistry [83]. While sensitivity for all adenocarcinoma is low, the subset of adenocarcinoma that are FDG-avid have a SUVmax that correlates with larger tumor size and increased depth of invasion [78].

Magnetic Resonance Imaging

Magnetic resonance imaging (MRI) is not routinely recommended as an imaging modality for the diagnosis or staging of gastric cancer. As an investigational imaging modality, MRI may be superior to CT for obtaining T stage of a gastric lesion, likely due to its soft tissue sensitivity [84]. This increased soft tissue resolution would make it ideal for radiomics. Indeed, a radiomics-generated nomogram has already demonstrated accuracy in predicting lymph node metastasis [85]. In addition, gadolinium-enhanced MRI has been shown to be beneficial for detecting liver metastasis [86]. Future directions of MRI research include development of radiomics for lymph node staging and combination MRI with FDG-PET. MRI has been shown to be beneficial in detection of peritoneal metastasis in comparison to CT, and does generate more accurate predictions of PCI score for appendiceal and colorectal carcinomatosis [87]. However, there is currently limited data on MRI detection of peritoneal metastasis in gastric cancer.

Staging Laparoscopy

Peritoneal metastasis is found on initial diagnosis in 14-17% of all patients diagnosed with gastric adenocarcinoma of any stage [88, 89], with up to 41% of diagnostic laparoscopies being positive for cancer cells [90]. Seeding of the peritoneal space with tumor cells is a complex molecular process that likely occurs via multiple mechanisms [91]. Both macroscopic peritoneal implants and cytologically discovered tumor cells bear the same prognostic significance, demonstrated by higher recurrence following curative-intent gastrectomy [92]. Thus, the diagnosis of peritoneal carcinomatosis is critical for prognosis and treatment in gastric cancer.

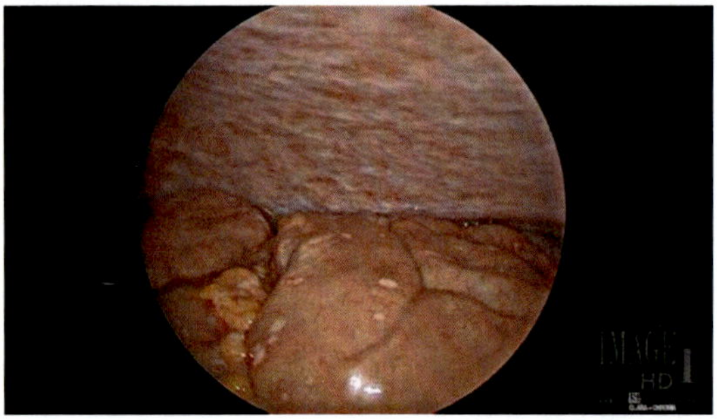

A

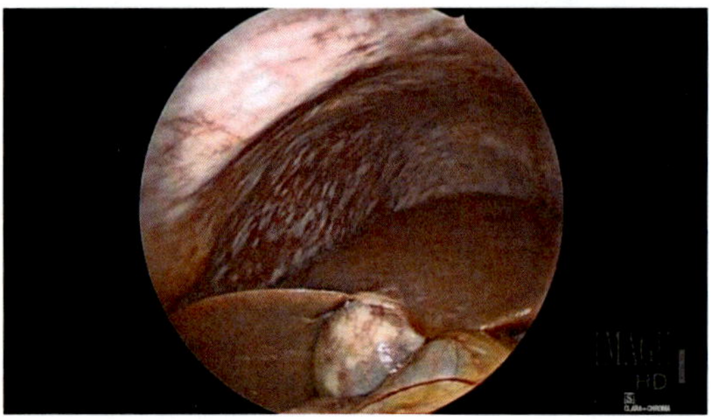

B

Figure 3. Laparoscopic images of peritoneal carcinomatosis on the (A) small bowel and (B) anterior parietal peritoneum.

The gold standard for staging of the peritoneum is laparoscopic visualization with cytopathologic analysis of peritoneal lavage fluid. Since the adoption of staging laparoscopy for gastric cancers the rate of non-therapeutic laparotomy has declined, with curative-intent gastrectomy reserved for patients free of macro- and microscopic peritoneal metastasis. Direct visualization of the peritoneal surfaces, as well as cytology obtained using peritoneal lavage, are sensitive and specific for diagnosing radiographically occult peritoneal disease (Figure 3) [93]. Peritoneal carcinomatosis index (PCI) score can be calculated, providing more prognostic data [94]. Despite its increasing adoption, laparoscopy still may be underutilized for staging potential surgical candidates [95]. Finally, many neoadjuvant chemotherapy protocols require diagnostic laparoscopy prior to and following neoadjuvant treatment [96].

Unfortunately, up to 29% of cytologically-negative patients who have undergone a R0 resection of their primary tumor still develop a peritoneal recurrence [97]. Compared with other diagnostic tests, staging laparoscopy is invasive and requires general anesthesia. Below we detail current practices and advancements in staging techniques for the detection of advanced disease.

Peritoneal Lavage

Laparoscopic inspection of the peritoneal surfaces alone can detect grossly visible tumor deposits but is insufficient to detect the presence of microscopic peritoneal tumor cells. With peritoneal lavage 50-100cc of saline is instilled into the peritoneum, aspirated, and sent for cytopathologic analysis. Positive cytology is defined as at least one positive adenocarcinoma cell by Papanicolaou stain. Patients with positive cytology demonstrate high rates of recurrence following curative resection [92]. Positive cytology, therefore, is considered a manifestation of metastatic disease. We routinely perform peritoneal lavage on all patients without signs of gross peritoneal involvement on diagnostic laparoscopy. Interestingly, among cytology-positive patients who undergo systemic chemotherapy, repeat staging laparoscopy showing conversion to cytology-negative has been associated with improved disease-free survival [98, 99]. Treating microscopic peritoneal metastasis may therefore be a rational strategy for this subset of patients with advanced cancer.

Molecular Assays

There is growing evidence that reverse transcription polymerase chain reaction (RT-PCR) detection of tumor-specific transcripts in RNA isolates from peritoneal lavage specimens is non-inferior, and possibly superior, to traditional cytology at detecting microscopic peritoneal metastatic cells [100]. RT-PCR is a rapid and objective technique requiring fewer cells for a positive test, thereby increasing the likelihood of detection of occult metastasis [101]. Several gene transcripts have been described as potential targets for amplification, but the most widely studied assay detects the presence of CEA mRNA [102]. Cytokeratin 20 (CK20), survivin, and MUC2 have also been evaluated [103]. Immunoassay for the CEA gene product appears to be inferior to nucleotide-based detection of the mRNA transcript [104].

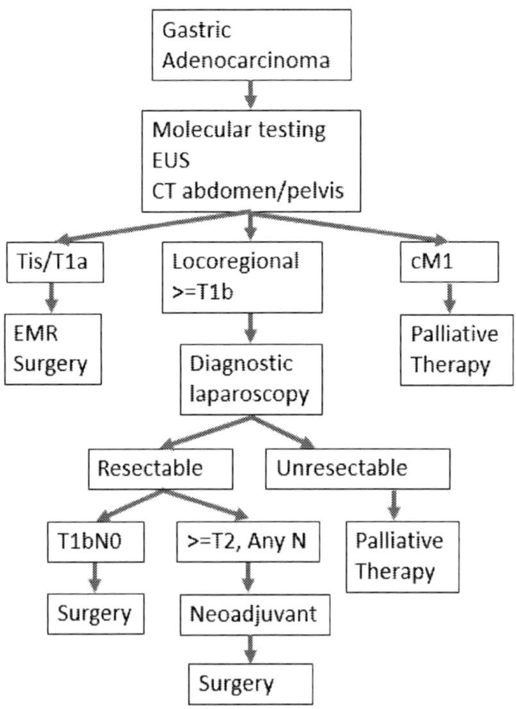

Figure 4. Algorithm for gastric adenocarcinoma diagnosis and staging.

RT-PCR for CEA in peritoneal lavage specimens may have prognostic significance. Wong et al., showed no difference in survival between patients whose lavage specimens were cytologically negative (CYT-) but RT-PCR positive (PCR+) and CYT+PCR+ [105]. Of patients who underwent R0 resection, those with preoperative lavage specimens that were PCR+ had a significantly worse disease-free survival than those whose specimens were PCR-. Criticisms of RT-PCR include increased cost, lack of standardization of specimen collection/processing, and false positive rate due to lymphocyte and mesothelial cell expression of CEA [106]. As such, cytology is still considered the diagnostic standard for occult peritoneal metastasis.

Conclusion

Diagnosis and staging of gastric adenocarcinoma present a challenge for clinicians due to late presentation and pattern of spread. Despite being the fifth most common cancer worldwide with several well-known risk factors, identifying at-risk patients can be difficult. For instance, gastric cancer incidence is not high enough to warrant a national screening program in most North American patients. When clinical symptoms do arise, the diagnosis can be easily missed or mistaken for benign disease, further contributing to delay in diagnosis. Once diagnosed, accurate staging tools are necessary. Though staging techniques have improved with the addition of laparoscopy, a proportion of patients inevitably will be over- or undertreated, likely leading to unnecessary morbidity and disease-specific mortality. Research in the early diagnosis and staging of gastric cancer focuses on increased accuracy in order to provide optimal therapy. Radiomics and molecular characterization of tumors both hold promise to improve patient selection for potential curative management. Standardization of RT-PCR for peritoneal lavage specimens should be considered, as evidence suggests that its accuracy exceeds that of traditional cytology. Finally, as clinical trials of targeted therapy and intraperitoneal chemotherapy progress, they will continue to depend on accurate staging to assess eligibility and response to therapy.

REFERENCES

[1] Anderson, W. F., et al., Age-specific trends in incidence of noncardia gastric cancer in US adults. *JAMA*, 2010. 303(17): p. 1723-8.

[2] Roder, D. M., The epidemiology of gastric cancer. *Gastric Cancer,* 2002. 5 Suppl 1: p. 5-11.

[3] Rawla, P. and A. Barsouk, Epidemiology of gastric cancer: global trends, risk factors and prevention. *Prz Gastroenterol,* 2019. 14(1): p. 26-38.

[4] Ajani, J. A., et al., Gastric adenocarcinoma. *Nat Rev Dis Primers,* 2017. 3: p. 17036.

[5] Oh, S. Y., et al., Natural History of Gastric Cancer: Observational Study of Gastric Cancer Patients Not Treated During Follow-Up. *Ann Surg Oncol*, 2019. 26(9): p. 2905-2911.

[6] Farag, S., et al., Revolutions in treatment options in gastrointestinal stromal tumours (GISTs): the latest updates. *Curr Treat Options* Oncol, 2020. 21(7): p. 55.

[7] Li, T. T., et al., Classification, clinicopathologic features and treatment of gastric neuroendocrine tumors. *World J Gastroenterol,* 2014. 20(1): p. 118-25.

[8] Bang, Y. J., et al., Trastuzumab in combination with chemotherapy versus chemotherapy alone for treatment of HER2-positive advanced gastric or gastro-oesophageal junction cancer (ToGA): a phase 3, open-label, randomised controlled trial. *The Lancet,* 2010. 376(9742): p. 687-697.

[9] Li, J., et al., Randomized, Double-Blind, Placebo-Controlled Phase III Trial of Apatinib in Patients With Chemotherapy-Refractory Advanced or Metastatic Adenocarcinoma of the Stomach or Gastroesophageal Junction. *J Clin Oncol*, 2016. 34(13): p. 1448-54.

[10] Akin Telli, T., et al., PD-1 and PD-L1 inhibitors in oesophago-gastric cancers. *Cancer Lett*, 2020. 469: p. 142-150.

[11] Maconi, G., G. Manes, and G. B. Porro, Role of symptoms in diagnosis and outcome of gastric cancer. *World J Gastroenterol*, 2008. 14(8): p. 1149-55.

[12] Kong, S. H., et al., Clinicopathologic features of asymptomatic gastric adenocarcinoma patients in Korea. *Jpn J Clin Oncol,* 2004. 34(1): p. 1-7.

[13] Axon, A., Symptoms and diagnosis of gastric cancer at early curable stage. *Best Pract Res Clin Gastroentero*l, 2006. 20(4): p. 697-708.

[14] Wanebo, H. J., et al., Cancer of the stomach. A patient care study by the American College of Surgeons. *Ann Surg,* 1993. 218(5): p. 583-92.

[15] Stephens, M. R., et al., Prognostic significance of alarm symptoms in patients with gastric cancer. *Br J Surg,* 2005. 92(7): p. 840-6.

[16] Moayyedi, P., et al., ACG and CAG Clinical Guideline: Management of Dyspepsia. *Am J Gastroenterol*, 2017. 112(7): p. 988-1013.

[17] Liou, J.-M., et al., The optimal age threshold for screening upper endoscopy for uninvestigated dyspepsia in Taiwan, an area with a higher prevalence of gastric cancer in young adults. *Gastrointestinal Endoscopy,* 2005. 61(7): p. 819-825.

[18] Guggenheim, D. E. and M. A. Shah, Gastric cancer epidemiology and risk factors. *J Surg Oncol*, 2013. 107(3): p. 230-6.

[19] Nolen, L. D., et al., Combating Gastric Cancer in Alaska Native People: An Expert and Community Symposium. *Gastroenterology,* 2020. 158(5): p. 1197-1201.

[20] Viacava, E. P. and G. T. Pack, Significance of supraclavicular signal node in patients with abdominal and thoracic cancer - A study of one hundred and twenty two cases. *Archives of Surgery,* 1944. 48(2): p. 109-119.

[21] Powell, F. C., et al., *Si*ster Mary Joseph's nodule: A clinical and histologic study. *Journal of the American Academy of Dermatology,* 1984. 10(4): p. 610-615.

[22] Fransen, G. A., et al., Meta-analysis: the diagnostic value of alarm symptoms for upper gastrointestinal malignancy. *Aliment Pharmacol Ther,* 2004. 20(10): p. 1045-52.

[23] Blumenthaler, A. N., et al., Relationship between initial management strategy and survival in patients with gastric outlet obstruction due to gastric cancer. *J Surg Oncol*, 2020.

[24] Shimada, H., et al., Clinical significance of serum tumor markers for gastric cancer: a systematic review of literature by the Task Force of the Japanese Gastric Cancer Association. *Gastric Cancer*, 2014. 17(1): p. 26-33.

[25] Lin, J. X., et al., Preoperative Tumor Markers Independently Predict Survival in Stage III Gastric Cancer Patients: Should We Include Tumor Markers in AJCC Staging? *Ann Surg Oncol*, 2018. 25(9): p. 2703-2712.

[26] Wang, W., et al., Prognostic significance of preoperative serum CA125, CA19-9 and CEA in gastric carcinoma. *Oncotarget,* 2016. 7(23): p. 35423-36.

[27] Suenaga, Y., et al., Prognostic significance of perioperative tumor marker levels in stage II/III gastric cancer. *World J Gastrointest* Oncol, 2019. 11(1): p. 17-27.

[28] El Abiad, R. and H. Gerke, Gastric cancer: endoscopic diagnosis and staging. *Surg Oncol Clin N Am*, 2012. 21(1): p. 1-19.

[29] Graham, D. Y., et al., Prospective evaluation of biopsy number in the diagnosis of esophageal and gastric carcinoma. *Gastroenterology,* 1982. 82(2): p. 228-231.

[30] Ballantyne, K. C., et al., Accuracy of identification of early gastric cancer. *Br J Surg,* 1987. 74(7): p. 618-9.

[31] Participants in the Paris, W., The Paris endoscopic classification of superficial neoplastic lesions: esophagus, stomach, and colon. *Gastrointestinal Endoscopy*, 2003. 58(6): p. S3-S43.

[32] Jung, K., et al., Borrmann Type 4 Advanced Gastric Cancer: Focus on the Development of Scirrhous Gastric Cancer. *Clin Endosc,* 2016. 49(4): p. 336-45.

[33] Ikoma, N., et al., Linitis Plastica: a Distinct Type of Gastric Cancer. *J Gastrointest Surg,* 2020. 24(5): p. 1018-1025.

[34] Blair, V. R., et al., Hereditary diffuse gastric cancer: updated clinical practice guidelines. *The Lancet Oncology*, 2020. 21(8): p. e386-e397.

[35] Kumar, S., et al., The role of endoscopy in the management of hereditary diffuse gastric cancer syndrome. *World J Gastroenterol,* 2019. 25(23): p. 2878-2886.

[36] Rudiger Siewert, J., et al., Adenocarcinoma of the esophagogastric junction: results of surgical therapy based on anatomical/ topographic classification in 1,002 consecutive patients. *Ann Surg,* 2000. 232(3): p. 353-61.

[37] Blot, W. J., Rising Incidence of Adenocarcinoma of the Esophagus and nGastric Cardia. *JAMA*: *The Journal of the American Medical Association,* 1991. 265(10).

[38] Lauren, P., The Two Histological Main Types of Gastric Carcinoma: Diffuse and So-Called Intestinal-Type Carcinoma. An Attempt at a Histo-Clinical Classification. *Acta Pathol Microbiol Scand*, 1965. 64: p. 31-49.

[39] Neumann, W. L., et al., Autoimmune atrophic gastritis--pathogenesis, pathology and management. *Nat Rev Gastroenterol Hepatol,* 2013. 10(9): p. 529-41.

[40] Schistosomes, liver flukes and Helicobacter pylori. IARC Working Group on the Evaluation of Carcinogenic Risks to Humans. Lyon, 7-14 June 1994. *IARC Monogr Eval Carcinog Risks Hum*, 1994. 61: p. 1-241.

[41] Qiu, M. Z., et al., Clinicopathological characteristics and prognostic analysis of Lauren classification in gastric adenocarcinoma in China. *J Transl Med,* 2013. 11: p. 58.

[42] Pernot, S., et al., Signet-ring cell carcinoma of the stomach: Impact on prognosis and specific therapeutic challenge. *World J Gastroenterol,* 2015. 21(40): p. 11428-38.

[43] Jacobs, M. F., et al., Outcomes of Endoscopic Surveillance in Individuals with Genetic Predisposition to Hereditary Diffuse Gastric Cancer. *Gastroenterology,* 2019. 157(1): p. 87-96.

[44] Roberts, M. E., et al., Comparison of CDH1 Penetrance Estimates in Clinically Ascertained Families vs Families Ascertained for Multiple Gastric Cancers. *JAMA Oncol,* 2019.

[45] Xicola, R. M., et al., Clinical features and cancer risk in families with pathogenic CDH1 variants irrespective of clinical criteria. *J Med Genet,* 2019. 56(12): p. 838-843.

[46] Cancer Genome Atlas Research, N., Comprehensive molecular characterization of gastric adenocarcinoma. *Nature,* 2014. 513(7517): p. 202-9.

[47] Cristescu, R., et al., Molecular analysis of gastric cancer identifies subtypes associated with distinct clinical outcomes. *Nat Med*, 2015. 21(5): p. 449-56.

[48] Fukayama, M. and T. Ushiku, Epstein-Barr virus-associated gastric carcinoma. *Pathol Res Pract,* 2011. 207(9): p. 529-37.

[49] Mathiak, M., et al., Clinicopathologic Characteristics of Microsatellite Instable Gastric Carcinomas Revisited: Urgent Need for Standardization. *Appl Immunohistochem Mol Morphol,* 2017. 25(1): p. 12-24.

[50] Rocken, C., Molecular classification of gastric cancer. *Expert Rev Mol Diagn*, 2017. 17(3): p. 293-301.

[51] Mazloom, A., et al., Role of Immune Checkpoint Inhibitors in Gastrointestinal Malignancies. *J Clin Med*, 2020. 9(8).

[52] Shitara, K., et al., Pembrolizumab versus paclitaxel for previously treated, advanced gastric or gastro-oesophageal junction cancer (KEYNOTE-061): a randomised, open-label, controlled, phase 3 trial. *The Lancet*, 2018. 392(10142): p. 123-133.

[53] Ohtsu, A., et al., Bevacizumab in combination with chemotherapy as first-line therapy in advanced gastric cancer: a randomized, double-blind, placebo-controlled phase III study. *J Clin Oncol,* 2011. 29(30): p. 3968-76.

[54] Pectasides, E., et al., Genomic Heterogeneity as a Barrier to Precision Medicine in Gastroesophageal Adenocarcinoma. *Cancer Discov*, 2018. 8(1): p. 37-48.
[55] Worthley, D. L., et al., Gastric adenocarcinoma and proximal polyposis of the stomach (GAPPS): a new autosomal dominant syndrome. *Gut,* 2012. 61(5): p. 774-9.
[56] Oliveira, C., et al., Familial gastric cancer: genetic susceptibility, pathology, and implications for management. *The Lancet Oncology,* 2015. 16(2): p. e60-e70.
[57] Ducimetiere, F., et al., Incidence of sarcoma histotypes and molecular subtypes in a prospective epidemiological study with central pathology review and molecular testing. *PLoS One*, 2011. 6(8): p. e20294.
[58] Gold, J. S., et al., Development and validation of a prognostic nomogram for recurrence-free survival after complete surgical resection of localised primary gastrointestinal stromal tumour: a retrospective analysis. *The Lancet Oncology*, 2009. 10(11): p. 1045-1052.
[59] Fletcher, C. D., et al., Diagnosis of gastrointestinal stromal tumors: A consensus approach. *Hum Pathol*, 2002. 33(5): p. 459-65.
[60] Ravegnini, G., et al., Pharmacogenetics in the treatment of gastrointestinal stromal tumors - an updated review. *Expert Opin Drug Metab Toxicol,* 2020. 16(9): p. 797-808.
[61] Thomas, D., et al., Long-term follow-up of a large series of patients with type 1 gastric carcinoid tumors: data from a multicenter study. *Eur J Endocrinol*, 2013. 168(2): p. 185-93.
[62] Sato, Y., et al., Management of gastric and duodenal neuroendocrine tumors. *World J Gastroenterol*, 2016. 22(30): p. 6817-28.
[63] Maehara, Y., et al., Postoperative outcome and sites of recurrence in patients following curative resection of gastric cancer. *Br J Surg,* 2000. 87(3): p. 353-7.
[64] Shi, X., et al., Development and validation of a nomogram to predict the prognosis of patients with gastric cardia cancer. *Sci Rep,* 2020. 10(1): p. 14143.

[65] Chen, Y., et al., A better prognostic stratification for the 8th edition of the AJCC staging system of gastric cancer by incorporating pT4aN0M0 into stage IIIA. *Surg Oncol*, 2019. 29: p. 90-96.

[66] Mocellin, S. and S. Pasquali, Diagnostic accuracy of endoscopic ultrasonography (EUS) for the preoperative locoregional staging of primary gastric cancer. *Cochrane Database Syst Rev*, 2015(2): p. CD009944.

[67] Power, D. G., et al., Endoscopic ultrasound can improve the selection for laparoscopy in patients with localized gastric cancer. *J Am Coll Surg*, 2009. 208(2): p. 173-8.

[68] Allen, C. J., et al., Staging laparoscopy and peritoneal cytology in patients with early stage gastric adenocarcinoma. *World J Surg* Oncol, 2020. 18(1): p. 39.

[69] Ajani, J. A., et al., *Gastric Cancer, Version 3.2016,* NCCN Clinical Practice Guidelines in Oncology. *J Natl Compr Canc Netw*, 2016. 14(10): p. 1286-1312.

[70] Kim, S. J., et al., Peritoneal metastasis: detection with 16- or 64-detector row CT in patients undergoing surgery for gastric cancer. *Radiology*, 2009. 253(2): p. 407-15.

[71] Guo, J.C., et al., Computed tomographic characteristics for patients with unresectable gastric cancer harboring low-volume peritoneal carcinomatosis. *Med Oncol*, 2017. 34(8): p. 143.

[72] Kim, M., et al., Gastric cancer: development and validation of a CT-based model to predict peritoneal metastasis. *Acta Radiol*, 2020. 61(6): p. 732-742.

[73] Liu, S., et al., Radiomics analysis using contrast-enhanced CT for preoperative prediction of occult peritoneal metastasis in advanced gastric cancer. *Eur Radiol*, 2020. 30(1): p. 239-246.

[74] Dong, D., et al., Development and validation of an individualized nomogram to identify occult peritoneal metastasis in patients with advanced gastric cancer. *Ann Oncol*, 2019. 30(3): p. 431-438.

[75] Chen, J., et al., Improvement in preoperative staging of gastric adenocarcinoma with positron emission tomography. *Cancer*, 2005. 103(11): p. 2383-90.

[76] Lehmann, K., et al., *(18)* FDG-PET-CT improves specificity of preoperative lymph-node staging in patients with intestinal but not diffuse-type esophagogastric adenocarcinoma. *Eur J Surg Oncol,* 2017. 43(1): p. 196-202.

[77] Choi, J. Y., et al., The clinical value of 18F-fluorodeoxyglucose uptake on positron emission tomography/computed tomography for predicting regional lymph node metastasis and non-curative surgery in primary gastric carcinoma. *Korean J Gastroenterol*, 2014. 64(6): p. 340-7.

[78] Oh, H. H., et al., The peak-standardized uptake value (P-SUV) by preoperative positron emission tomography-computed tomography (PET-CT) is a useful indicator of lymph node metastasis in gastric cancer. *J Surg Oncol,* 2011. 104(5): p. 530-3.

[79] Smyth, E., et al., A prospective evaluation of the utility of 2-deoxy-2-[(18) F]fluoro-D-glucose positron emission tomography and computed tomography in staging locally advanced gastric cancer. *Cancer*, 2012. 118(22): p. 5481-8.

[80] Yoshioka, T., et al., Evaluation of 18F-FDG PET in patients with advanced, metastatic, or recurrent gastric cancer. *J Nucl Med,* 2003. 44(5): p. 690-9.

[81] Stahl, A., et al., FDG PET imaging of locally advanced gastric carcinomas: correlation with endoscopic and histopathological findings. *Eur J Nucl Med Mol Imaging,* 2003. 30(2): p. 288-95.

[82] Alakus, H., et al., Variable 18F-fluorodeoxyglucose uptake in gastric cancer is associated with different levels of GLUT-1 expression. *Nucl Med Commun,* 2010. 31(6): p. 532-8.

[83] Kaneko, Y., et al., Improving patient selection for 18F-FDG PET scanning in the staging of gastric cancer. *J Nucl Med*, 2015. 56(4): p. 523-9.

[84] Borggreve, A. S., et al., Imaging strategies in the management of gastric cancer: current role and future potential of MRI. *Br J Radiol,* 2019. 92(1097): p. 20181044.

[85] Chen, W., et al., Evaluation of Lymph Node Metastasis in Advanced Gastric Cancer Using Magnetic Resonance Imaging-Based Radiomics. *Front Oncol,* 2019. 9: p. 1265.

[86] Wang, Z. and J. Q. Chen, Imaging in assessing hepatic and peritoneal metastases of gastric cancer: a systematic review. *BMC Gastroenterol*, 2011. 11: p. 19.

[87] Low, R. N. and R. M. Barone, *Imaging for Peritoneal Metastases. Surg Oncol Clin N Am*, 2018. 27(3): p. 425-442.

[88] Thomassen, I., et al., Peritoneal carcinomatosis of gastric origin: a population-based study on incidence, survival and risk factors. *Int J Cancer*, 2014. 134(3): p. 622-8.

[89] Gretschel, S., et al., Surgical strategies for gastric cancer with synchronous peritoneal carcinomatosis. *Br J Surg*, 2006. 93(12): p. 1530-5.

[90] Ribeiro, U., Prognostic significance of intraperitoneal free cancer cells obtained by laparoscopic peritoneal lavage in patients with gastric cancer. *Journal of Gastrointestinal Surgery*, 1998. 2(3): p. 244-249.

[91] Sun, F., M. Feng, and W. Guan, Mechanisms of peritoneal dissemination in gastric cancer. *Oncol Lett,* 2017. 14(6): p. 6991-6998.

[92] Bentrem, D., et al., The value of peritoneal cytology as a preoperative predictor in patients with gastric carcinoma undergoing a curative resection. *Ann Surg Oncol*, 2005. 12(5): p. 347-53.

[93] Ramos, R. F., et al., Staging laparoscopy in gastric cancer to detect peritoneal metastases: A systematic review and meta-analysis. *Eur J Surg Oncol,* 2016. 42(9): p. 1315-21.

[94] Yarema, R., et al., Gastric cancer with peritoneal metastases: Efficiency of standard treatment methods. *World J Gastrointest Oncol,* 2020. 12(5): p. 569-581.

[95] Groh, E. M., et al., Staging Laparoscopy is Underutilized in the Management of Gastric Adenocarcinoma. *Ann Surg Oncol*, 2020. 27(5): p. 1473-1479.

[96] Cardona, K., et al., Role of repeat staging laparoscopy in locoregionally advanced gastric or gastroesophageal cancer after neoadjuvant therapy. *Ann Surg Oncol,* 2013. 20(2): p. 548-54.

[97] D'Angelica, M., et al., Patterns of initial recurrence in completely resected gastric adenocarcinoma. *Ann Surg,* 2004. 240(5): p. 808-16.

[98] Mezhir, J. J., et al., Positive peritoneal cytology in patients with gastric cancer: natural history and outcome of 291 patients. *Ann Surg Oncol*, 2010. 17(12): p. 3173-80.

[99] Jamel, S., et al., Prognostic significance of peritoneal lavage cytology in staging gastric cancer: systematic review and meta-analysis. *Gastric Cancer*, 2018. 21(1): p. 10-18.

[100] Kolomanska, M. M. and S. Gluszek, Free cancer cells in gastric cancer - methods of detection, clinical and prognostic importance (meta-analysis). *Contemp Oncol* (Pozn), 2020. 24(1): p. 67-74.

[101] Tokuda, K., et al., Clinical significance of CEA-mRNA expression in peritoneal lavage fluid from patients with gastric cancer. *International Journal of Molecular Medicine*, 2003.

[102] Chae, H. D., Role of genetic detection in peritoneal washes with gastric carcinoma: The past, present and future. *World J Gastrointest Oncol*, 2016. 8(3): p. 289-96.

[103] Dalal, K. M., et al., Detection of micrometastases in peritoneal washings of gastric cancer patients by the reverse transcriptase polymerase chain reaction. *Gastric Cancer,* 2008. 11(4): p. 206-13.

[104] Wang, J. Y., et al., Gastric cancer cell detection in peritoneal lavage: RT-PCR for carcinoembryonic antigen transcripts versus the combined cytology with peritoneal carcinoembryonic antigen levels. *Cancer Lett,* 2005. 223(1): p. 129-35.

[105] Wong, J., et al., Rt-PCR increases detection of submicroscopic peritoneal metastases in gastric cancer and has prognostic significance. *J Gastrointest Surg*, 2012. 16(5): p. 889-96; discussion 896.

[106] Kodera, Y., et al., Quantitative detection of disseminated free cancer cells in peritoneal washes with real-time reverse transcriptase-

polymerase chain reaction: a sensitive predictor of outcome for patients with gastric carcinoma. *Ann Surg*, 2002. 235(4): p. 499-506.

Image Sources

Ajani, J. A., et al., Gastric adenocarcinoma. *Nat Rev Dis Primers*, 2017. 3: p. 17036.

Maeda, E., et al., Characteristic waffle-like appearance of gastric linitis plastica: A case report. *Oncol Lett,* 2015. 9(1): p. 262-264.

Yoshinaga, S., et al., Clinical impact of endoscopic submucosal dissection for superficial adenocarcinoma located at the esophagogastric junction. *Gastrointest Endosc*, 2008. 67(2): p. 202-9.

Silva, J. C., et al., Bleeding malignant gastric ulcer: successful endoscopic hemostasis with an over-the-scope clip. *VideoGIE,* 2020. 5(4): p. 146-147.

Lee, H. H., et al., Low accuracy of endoscopic ultrasonography for detailed T staging in gastric cancer. *World J Surg Oncol*, 2012. 10: p. 190.

In: Gastric Peritoneal Carcinomatosis
Editors: F. López Mozos et al.
ISBN: 978-1-53619-487-6

Chapter 4

HISTOPATHOLOGICAL AND MOLECULAR CLASSIFICATIONS OF GASTRIC CANCER

***Carolina Martinez-Ciarpaglini*[1-3,*], *Clara Alfaro-Cervelló*[1-3], *Lorena Alarcon*[1] *and Tania Fleitas*[2]**

[1]Department of Pathology, Hospital Clinico Universitario of Valencia, Biomedical Institute INCLIVA

[2]Department of Medical Oncology, Hospital Clinico Universitario of Valencia, Biomedical Institute INCLIVA

[3]Departement of Pathology, University of Valencia

ABSTRACT

The development of a solid and reproducible pathohistological classification system is crucial not only for diagnosis but also to make patient-specific decisions regarding treatment. In gastric cancer, several histopathological classifications have been proposed but the most common and worldwide used are the Lauren and the World Health

* Corresponding Author's E-mail: carolaciarpaglini@gmail.com.

Organization (WHO) classifications. Lauren`s classification introduced in 1965, divided the histology of gastric cancer into two groups, the intestinal type, and the diffuse type. The World Health Organization (WHO) classification issued in 2010, appears to be the most detailed and divided gastric cancer into several sub-groups including poorly cohesive papillary, tubular, mucinous, and mixed carcinoma. However, morphology has a limited utility in terms of predicting the molecular heterogeneity characteristic of gastric cancer. In recent years, molecular methods such as next-generation sequencing (NGS) including deoxyribonucleic acid (DNA) sequencing, ribonucleic acid (RNA) sequencing, whole-exome sequencing, copy number variation analysis, and DNA methylation arrays have been used to classify human tumors into molecular subtypes. Significant advances in the understanding of gastric cancer have been achieved as a result of comprehensive molecular and functional characterizations such as The Cancer Genome Atlas (TCGA) classification and Asian Cancer Research Group (ACRG) Subtypes. TGCA classification is a multi-omic-based classification established four main subgroups of gastric cancer: tumors positive for Epstein-Barr virus (EBV-GC), microsatellite unstable tumors (MSI-GC), genomic stable tumors, and tumors with chromosomal instability. The ARCG classification established four subtypes based on mRNA expression: microsatellite unstable high (MSI-high), microsatellite stable/epithelial-mesenchymal transition (MSS/EMT), microsatellite stable/epithelial/TP53 intact (MSS/TP53+), and microsatellite stable/epithelial/TP53 loss (MSS/TP53-). In this chapter, we will detail the histopathological and molecular classifications of gastric cancer and their clinical applicability.

INTRODUCTION

Correct classification of epithelial neoplasms into biologically rational entities is the basis for the proper understanding of the pathogenesis of the disease, its epidemiology, and clinical management. The development of a solid and reproducible pathohistological classification system is crucial not only for diagnosis but also to make patient-specific decisions regarding treatment.

Gastric cancer is a heterogeneous disease with different phenotypes, genotypes, and clinical progress, including sensitivity to treatments and prognosis. Familial aggregation explains around 10% of cases and 1-3% of all gastric cancers are associated with inherited genetic predisposition disorders, such as familial adenomatous polyposis (APC mutation), hereditary diffuse gastric cancer (*CDH1* mutations/loss of heterozygosity), and gastric adenocarcinoma and proximal polyposis of the stomach (GAPPS) [1, 2]. However, most sporadic gastric cancers are now considered to be inflammation-driven and their etiology is characteristically environmental, usually related to *H. pylori* infection [3]. Chronic *H. pylori* infection is recognized as the main cause of non-cardia (distal) gastric cancer (odds ratio 5.9 within 10 years of infection) [4]. Patients with gastric intestinal metaplasia (GIM) may have a greater than a tenfold increased risk of gastric cancer than the general population and the more extensive GIM correlates with increased gastric adenocarcinoma risk (especially if it extends to the body) [5, 6]. Gastric dysplasia is linked to an increased risk of adenocarcinoma (6% of patients with high-grade dysplasia progress to cancer within 5 years) and should alert to the possibility of synchronous gastric cancer [6].

5-10% of gastric carcinomas are associated with Epstein-Barr virus (EBV) infection, especially in tumors located in the cardia and gastric pouch [7, 8]. Smoking is associated with an increased risk of both gastric cardia (HR, 2.86; 95% CI, 1.73e4.70) and non-cardia (HR, 2.04; 95% CI, 1.32e3.16) cancers [9]. Heavy alcohol drinking has been pointed to as a risk factor for gastric cancer; however, the available information on the association between alcohol consumption and risk of gastric cancer is contradictory [9, 10]. Other proposed risk factors are diet (salt, preserved meats, coffee), low socioeconomic status, obesity (body mass index over 25 kg/m is associated with 1.13 odds ratio of developing cancer), pernicious anemia (risk of gastric cancer 6.9%), previous gastric surgery, race/ethnicity (higher risk in Asians and African Americans) and blood group A, among others [2].

These multiple heterogeneities reflects also in the morphological diversity of gastric cancer. For this reason, several histopathological classifications have been advocated: the classifications according to Lauren [11], Ming [12], the World Health Organization (WHO) [13], Nakamura et al. [14], Mulligan [15], Goseki et al. [16], and Carneiro [17], as well as the

Japanese classification [17]. The most common and worldwide used are the Lauren and the WHO classifications. Lauren`s classification, introduced in 1965, divided the histology of gastric cancer into two groups: the intestinal type and the diffuse type. The WHO classification issued in 2010 appears to be the most detailed and divided gastric cancer into several sub-groups including poorly cohesive, papillary, tubular, mucinous, and mixed carcinoma. Both classifications, the Lauren`s and the WHO, are however similar and their categories correspond to each other as we will discuss later in this chapter.

Although the morphology is the base for diagnosis in routine practice, it has a limited utility in terms of predicting the molecular heterogeneity characteristic of gastric cancer. In recent years, molecular methods such as next-generation sequencing (NGS) including deoxyribonucleic acid (DNA) sequencing, ribonucleic acid (RNA) sequencing, whole-exome sequencing, copy number variation (CNV) analysis, and DNA methylation arrays have been used to classify human tumors into molecular subtypes. Significant advances in the understanding of gastric cancer have been achieved as a result of comprehensive molecular and functional characterizations such as The Cancer Genome Atlas (TCGA) classification and The Asian Cancer Research Group (ACRG) Subtypes [18, 19]. TGCA classification is a multi-omic-based classification that established four main subgroups of gastric cancer: tumors positive for Epstein-Barr virus (EBV-GC), microsatellite unstable tumors (MSI-GC), genomic stable tumors, and tumors with chromosomal instability. The ARCG classification established four subtypes based on mRNA expression: microsatellite unstable high (MSI-high), microsatellite stable/epithelial-mesenchymal transition (MSS/EMT), microsatellite stable/epithelial/TP53 intact (MSS/TP53+), and microsatellite stable/epithelial/TP53 loss (MSS/TP53-). In this chapter, we will detail the histopathological and molecular classifications of gastric cancer and their clinical applicability.

Histopathological Classification of Gastric Cancer

Lauren's Classification

Lauren's classification is the most practical, useful, and widely applicable histopathological classification system in gastric cancer. This classification was proposed by Lauren in 1965 by observations based only on the microscopical morphology of tumors [11]. According to Lauren's classification, gastric adenocarcinomas are divided into diffuse and intestinal types (Table 1). The last term was coined at least 15 years before Lauren's publication by some authors who suggested that many cases of gastric carcinomas arise from intestinal metaplasia in the stomach. A mixed subtype composed of both intestinal and diffuse components and an undifferentiated subtype was included posteriorly in the classification.

Table 1. Lauren classification of gastric cancer

• Diffuse type: – Lack of or poor cohesion between the neoplastic cells – Composed of scattered, small clusters or rows of cells with little or no gland formation – Neoplastic cells usually show an atypical morphology with irregular nuclear contours and variable amounts of eosinophilic cytoplasm – In some cases, there is a variable component of cells showing the so-called signet ring morphology – Signet ring cells show ample cytoplasmic mucin, which appears optically clear on H&E staining and an eccentrically placed nucleus – Diffuse gastric cancer is characterized by an infiltrative growth pattern knows as "linitis plastica".
• Intestinal type: – Composed of tubular or glandular structures similar to intestinal adenocarcinoma – Neoplastic cells usually contain apical mucin vacuoles – Unlike diffuse gastric cancer, intestinal tumors grow along broad cohesive fronts to form an exophytic mass
• Mixed
• Undifferentiated

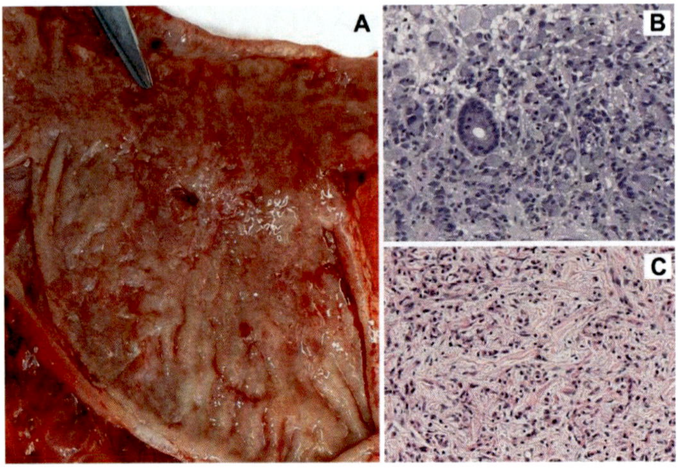

Figure 1. Macroscopic and microscopic findings in diffuse gastric carcinoma.
A. Linitis plastica pattern: note the diffuse rugal flattening and a rigid thickened wall.
B. Signet ring cells show large mucin vacuoles that fulfill and expand the cytoplasm and push the nucleus to the periphery C. In some cases, the cells show no signet ring-cell morphology, instead, they show an atypical morphology with irregular nuclear contours and variable amounts of eosinophilic cytoplasm. This type of neoplasm corresponds to the "poorly cohesive no otherwise specified" category of the WHO classification.

The main characteristic of the diffuse gastric cancer type is the lack or the poorly cohesion between the neoplastic cells. This type of tumor is composed of scattered, small clusters or rows of cells with little or no gland formation (Figure 1). The neoplastic cells usually show an atypical morphology with irregular nuclear contours and variable amounts of eosinophilic cytoplasm. This type of neoplasm corresponds to the "poorly cohesive not otherwise specified" category of the WHO classification (see section 1.2). In some cases, there is a variable component of cells showing the so-called "signet ring" morphology (Figure 1b). Signet ring cells show large mucin vacuoles that fulfill and expand the cytoplasm and push the nucleus to the periphery. Diffuse gastric cancer may show a variable component of signet ring cells. Tumors composed exclusively or predominantly of signet ring cells correspond to the "poorly cohesive signet ring cell type" category of the WHO classification (see section 1.2).

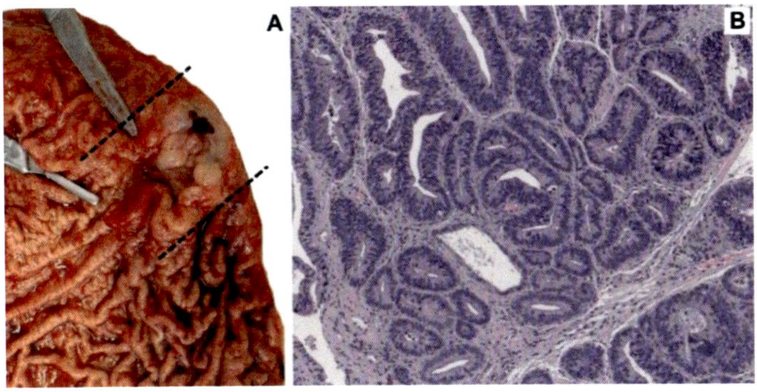

Figure 2. Macroscopic and microscopic findings in gastric carcinoma intestinal-subtype. A. Unlike diffuse gastric cancer, intestinal tumors grow along broad cohesive fronts to form an exophytic mass. B The ***intestinal-type gastric cancer*** is composed of tubular or glandular structures similar to intestinal adenocarcinoma. The neoplastic cells in this type of tumor are atypical and usually contain apical mucin vacuoles.

The intestinal-type gastric cancer is composed of tubular or glandular structures similar to intestinal adenocarcinoma (Figure 2). The neoplastic cells in this type of tumor are atypical and usually contain apical mucin vacuoles. Unlike diffuse gastric cancer, intestinal tumors grow along broad cohesive fronts to form an exophytic mass. Intestinal gastric cancer in Lauren´s classification corresponds to the "tubular gastric cancer category" of the WHO classification of gastric cancer tumors.

Typically, gastric cancer presents as a mass lesion; in other cases, a nonhealing gastric ulcer may be the presenting form [2]. Diffuse gastric cancer is characterized by an infiltrative growth pattern knows as "linitis plastic." In these cases, neoplastic cells permeate deeply through the gastric wall, evoking an intense desmoplastic reaction causing diffuse rugal flattening and a rigid thickened wall. The pattern of linitis plastica is highly correlated with the presence of signet ring cells [20].

In 2011, three subtypes of gastric cancer were proposed by Shah et al. based on tumor location and histological features, the so-called Modified Lauren´s Classification (Table 2) [21]. This proposal established 3 scenarios based not only on the histological appearance of the lesion but also on tumor location and association with pre-existing atrophy in the surrounding mucosa:

- *Proximal non-diffuse gastric cancer*: Comprises tumors located in the gastric cardia or gastroesophageal junction. This category includes intestinal tumors with any grade of differentiation or mixed tumors with a minor component of diffuse carcinoma. The surrounding mucosa usually evidence of glandular dysplasia in the setting of chronic inflammation without atrophy.
- *Diffuse Gastric Cancer:* This category includes exclusively tumors composed entirely by diffuse morphology located anywhere in the stomach. Mucinous tumors (from the WHO classification) should not be included. In these cases, the remaining non-tumoral mucosa shows no apparent gastritis or atrophy.
- *Distal non-diffuse Gastric Cancer*: In these cases, the bulk of the tumor is usually located in the distal stomach and may extend to the midbody or the pylorus. This category includes intestinal tumors with any grade of differentiation or mixed tumors with a minor component of diffuse carcinoma.

Table 2. Modified Lauren´s Classification of gastric cancer

• Proximal non-diffuse gastric cancer: – Comprises tumors located in the gastric cardia or gastroesophageal junction – Includes intestinal tumors with any grade of differentiation or mixed tumors with a minor component of diffuse carcinoma – Surrounding mucosa usually shows evidence of glandular dysplasia in the setting of chronic inflammation without atrophy
• Diffuse gastric cancer: – Includes tumors composed entirely of diffuse morphology located anywhere in the stomach – In these cases, the remaining nontumoral mucosa shows no apparent gastritis or atrophy
• Distal non-diffuse Gastric Cancer: – In these cases, the bulk of the tumor is usually located in the distal stomach and may extend to the midbody or the pylorus – This category includes intestinal tumors with any grade of differentiation or mixed tumors with a minor component of diffuse carcinoma

The WHO Classification

The WHO classification of gastric tumors comprises a more detailed classification of various sub-groups based on morphological and in some cases immune expression profiles of tumors (Table 3).

Table 3. WHO classification of gastric cancer

- Tubular adenocarcinoma (well, moderately and poorly differentiated)
- Poorly cohesive carcinoma, signet-ring cell phenotype
- Poorly cohesive carcinoma, NOS.
- Adenocarcinoma with mixed subtypes
- Papillary adenocarcinoma
- Micropapillary carcinoma
- Mucinous adenocarcinoma
- Hepatoid adenocarcinoma
- Adenosquamous carcinoma
- Squamous cell carcinoma
- Undifferentiated carcinoma
- Carcinoma with lymphoid stroma
- Adenocarcinoma with enteroblastic differentiation
- Adenocarcinoma of fundic gland type

Main similarities and differences between Lauren and WHO classifications of gastric cancer are:

- WHO classification separates tubular gastric carcinoma into 3 categories: well, moderately, and poorly differentiated, based on tubular formation.
- Lauren's intestinal subtype corresponds with the papillary and the well and moderately differentiated tubular categories of the WHO classification.
- Lauren diffuse subtype corresponds with the poorly cohesive category of the WHO classification [20].
- WHO classification separates poorly cohesive carcinoma into two categories [20].

   - Poorly cohesive, signet ring cell phenotype: composed only or predominately (more than 90%) of signet ring cells
   - Poorly cohesive, not otherwise specified (NOS): all other cases that do not display signet ring cell morphology.
- Both classifications recognize a mixed subtype, usually composed of cases with intestinal/tubular or papillary and diffuse/poorly cohesive components.
- There is currently no cutoff concerning the percentage of each component for a tumor to be classified as mixed adenocarcinoma.
- Most of the undifferentiated cases in the Lauren classification comprise cases classified as poorly differentiated tubular adenocarcinomas according to the WHO classification.
- WHO classification includes a series of less frequent variants, such as papillary, hepatoid, lymphoid stroma rich, among others, which are not defined in the Lauren classification.

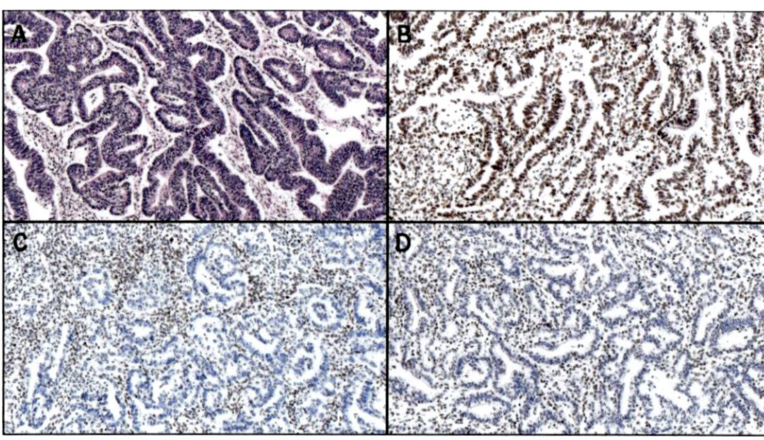

Figure 3. Microsatellite unstable gastric carcinoma, intestinal subtype. A. Tumor cells forming tubular structures, reminiscent intestinal carcinoma. B. Nuclear MHS6 expression is preserved in all tumor cells. Note the complete loss of nuclear staining for MLH1 (C) and PMS2 (D) in all tumor cells, with positive internal control in Peritumorous lymphocytes and stromal cells.

Prognostic Relevance of the Histopathological Classifications

In some studies, Lauren`s pathohistological subtype was an independent prognostic factor in gastric cancer patients undergoing gastrectomy in which patients with intestinal-type gastric cancer had a better 5-year overall survival than diffuse type and mixed type (43.4%, $P < 0.001$) [22]. Moreover, Lauren's subtype seems to predict survival and response to chemotherapy [23–25]. However, the results of other studies do not support this idea [26, 27]. The Modified Lauren's classification seems to represent a more reliable prognostic factor for gastric cancer patients with gastrectomy [28].

There is some evidence supporting the association between some histopathological subtypes of gastric cancer in the WHO classification and prognosis. However, in clinical practice, particularly as far as survival is concerned, all classifications of gastric cancer are of limited significance so far. The clinical-stage of GCA, independent of cancer type, is the most important single and independent factor that determines survival. The 5-year survival rate of early gastric cancer can reach > 95% [29]. For patients undergoing resection surgery, the 5-year survival rate is around 20-40%, whereas, in non-operated patients, it is 3–5% [30].

Microsatellite instability (MSI) in gastric cancer is associated with a better outcome [3, 7, 31].

The prognostic relevance of the morphological classifications of gastric cancer is still controversial, probably because of the high heterogeneity, lack of standardization, or the low reproducibility of the histopathological criteria [27, 32, 33]. Modified Lauren classification according to tumor location seems to improve the prognostic value [28].

Immunohistochemical Studies and Ancillary Techniques

Although the systematic immunohistochemical study is not routinely performed nor necessary in all cases, in some instances it may be necessary to establish the differential diagnosis with metastatic carcinoma from other organs.

Gastric carcinomas express cytokeratin (CK) 7 (CK7) in around 50-70%, CK20 in 30-48%, and CDX in 60% of cases [34, 35]. Low weigh CK such as CK5/6 may be expressed in around 15% of cases [35].

The patterns of mucins expression in GC is very variable, ranging from intestinal to gastric type. MUC is expressed in 30% and MUC5A in 70% of cases [34, 35].

E-cadherin or cytokeratin subtyping does not aid in the identification of signet ring cells [32].

Microsatellite instability (MSI) is detected in 15-30% of all gastric carcinomas [7, 36]. For the evaluation of MSI, most of the published studies follow the international consensus meeting proposed in 1997, the 'Bethesda panel,' which recommends the use of five markers for the uniform analysis of MSI in CRC [37]. These included two mononucleotide repeats (BAT-25 and BAT-26) and three dinucleotides (D5S346, D2S123, and D17S250) repeats. However, the sensitivity and specificity of this panel were questioned in the revised Bethesda guidelines for Lynch syndrome [38]. Dinucleotide repeats are also highly polymorphic, and their use in MSI screening requires the analysis of the corresponding normal tissue. For all these reasons, the revised Bethesda guidelines recommend the addition of more mononucleotide markers and highlight the need for further validation of MSI testing in tumor types other than colorectal and endometrial carcinoma. The description of quasi-monomorphic mononucleotides, showing a homozygous or quasi-homozygous state, with only minor size variations, allowed the MSI study in the absence of matching normal DNA. From these, NR-21 seems to be the most efficient marker, constantly unstable in all MSI tumors by PCR.

For the MSI status determination, the agreement between the immunohistochemical study and the polymerase chain reaction (PCR) for the MSI status in gastric cancer is excellent, and as in colorectal cancer, the PCR may be used only when the immunohistochemistry is not conclusive [7]. To performed a correct evaluation, only nuclear staining with or without cytoplasmic staining in tumor cells should be considered positive.

Peritumorous lymphocytes, stromal cells, and non-neoplastic epithelial cells should be used as internal control. Only the complete loss of nuclear staining with positive internal control should be considered as loss of mismatch repair (MMR) protein expression. The normal expression is defined as the presence of nuclear staining in tumor cells, irrespective of the intensity.

EBV can be demonstrated in 1.8-18% of all sporadic gastric carcinomas [39]. EBV expression in gastric cancer is strongly associated with the gastric carcinoma with lymphoid stroma variant of the WHO classification [40] (Figure 4) EBV encoded RNA (EBER) in situ hybridization is the most sensitive method for detecting EBV in paraffin-embedded tissues and stains all tumor cells [41, 42].

Differential Diagnosis With Metastatic Lobular Breast Carcinoma

Breast carcinoma is the third most frequent source of metastasis to the stomach (14%) [43]. Interestingly, the vast majority of breast carcinomas metastatic to the stomach belong to the lobular subtype (97%) [44].

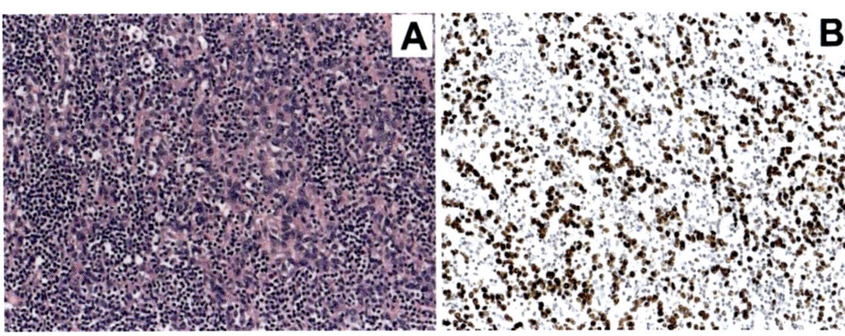

Figure 4. Epstein-Baar virus expression in gastric carcinoma with lymphoid stroma subtype. A. Neoplastic cells are arranged primarily in microalveolar, thin trabecular, and primitive tubular patterns uniformly distributed throughout a dense lymphoid stroma. B. In situ hybridization study for EBER is intensely and diffusely positive in all tumor cells.

The most common macroscopic growth pattern of presentation of metastatic breast carcinoma to the stomach is linitis plastica, indistinguishable from primary diffuse carcinoma [45]. Morphologically, metastatic lobular breast carcinoma shows poorly cohesive, round tumor cells arranged in linear cords between the normal gastric glands, very similar to primary diffuse carcinoma [35, 45].

Estrogen receptor (ER), progesterone receptor (PR), and GCDFP-15 are highly specific for metastatic breast carcinomas, whereas CK20 and CDX2 are highly specific for primary gastric carcinomas [45]. The combination of ER, PR, and GCDFP-15 help distinguish primary gastric carcinomas (consistently negative) from metastatic breast carcinomas (usually positive) [35]. GATA3 is rarely expressed (around 10% of cases) [46].

Loss of E-cadherin is not useful for the differential diagnosis, as it occurs in both invasive lobular carcinoma of the breast and primary diffuse gastric carcinoma [45].

Differential Diagnosis With Metastatic Lobular Breast Carcinoma

Malignant melanoma is the tumor that most frequently metastasized to the stomach (27% of all metastatic tumors in the stomach), followed by lung cancer (19%) [43]. Most melanomas found in the gastrointestinal tract are metastatic and a small proportion (around 4%) are primary mucosal melanomas [47].

Microscopic preoperative diagnosis of gastric melanoma may be a challenge and relies on the identification of melanin pigment [48].

Some gastric melanoma may present poorly cohesive epithelioid cells resembling a primary diffuse carcinoma. High pleomorphism, prominent nucleoli, and nuclear inclusions may suggest a melanoma, especially in the absence of melanic deposition [48]. S100, tyrosinase, MelanA, HMB45, and SOX10 are useful to demonstrate the melanic nature of tumor cells, especially in nonpigmented cases [47, 49].

Molecular Classification of Gastric Cancer

Molecular profiling of GC allows a better understanding of its pathogenesis and prognosis and can contribute to the development of targeted therapies in the era of personalized medicine. There are currently two proposed GC molecular classifications, established as part of The Cancer Genome Atlas (TCGA) project and by the Asian Cancer Research Group (ACRG) [18, 19]. As described for the different histological classifications, molecular subtypes are partially overlapping.

The Cancer Genome Atlas (TCGA) Classification

The TCGA project analyzed 295 primary gastric adenocarcinomas not treated with prior chemotherapy or radiotherapy and collected from various world regions. Several molecular platforms were used, including whole-exome sequencing, whole-genome sequencing, copy number analysis, DNA methylation profiling, messenger RNA sequencing, microRNA sequencing, reverse-phase protein array, and MSI testing. This multi-omics approach identified four major molecular subtypes: tumors positive for Epstein–Barr virus (EBV-GC) (~9%), tumors with microsatellite instability (MSI-GC) (~22%), genomically stable tumors (~20%), and tumors with chromosomal instability (CIN) (~50%). Although all subtypes were found throughout the stomach, some preferential locations were found. No survival differences between the four subgroups were found in the initial report.

Tumors positive for EBV are more frequently found in male patients, located in the gastric fundus or body. These tumors showed intense DNA promoter hypermethylation, including CDKN2A (p16INK4A), but lacked MLH1 hypermethylation characteristic of MSI. EBV-positive tumors also showed recurrent PIK3CA mutations, as well as ARID1A and BCOR mutations. Other alterations include amplification of JAK2, ERBB2 (HER2), programmed death-1 receptor ligand 1 (PD-L1), and PD-L2, the latter correlating with immunohistochemical overexpression.

Table 4. TCGA molecular classification

- EBV positive
  - Male patients
  - Gastric fundus or body
  - DNA promoter hypermethylation
  - PIK3CA mutations
  - PD-L1 and PD-L2 amplification
- MSI
  - Older patients
  - Antrum
  - Intestinal histology
  - Hypermethylation of MLH1
- Genomically stable
  - Younger patients
  - Distal stomach
  - Diffuse histology
  - Low mutational burden and copy number alterations.
- Chromosomal instability
  - Gastroesophageal junction or cardia
  - Intestinal histology
  - Marked aneuploidy and highly variable chromosomal copy number
  - Mutations of TP53.
  - Amplification of EGFR, ERBB2 (HER2), ERBB3, FGFR2, MET, VEGFA, and KRAS/NRAS.

Tumors with MSI develop in the elderly and are mainly located in the antrum. Tumors with MSI are associated with intestinal histology. MSI is a genetic alteration consisting of repetitive short nucleotide sequences (microsatellites), depending on the inactivation of DNA MMR activity. Four genes play a critical role in MMR activity: MLH1 (mutL homologue 1), MSH2 (mutS homologue 2), MSH6 (mutS homologue 6) and PMS2 (postmeiotic segregation increased 2). MSI-positive gastric cancer frequently shows hypermethylation of MLH1 [50]. These cases generally lacked targetable amplifications but showed elevated mutation rates in PIK3CA, ERBB3, ERBB2, and EGFR. As in colorectal adenocarcinoma, MSI can be related to Lynch syndrome. However, in contrast to MSI colorectal adenocarcinoma, there is no association with BRAF mutations.

Genomically stable tumors are diagnosed at a younger age and are distally located. Histologically, they are enriched in the diffuse histological type and have the worst prognosis among the four TCGA subtypes. These tumors are characterized by a low mutational burden and copy number alterations. Molecular alterations include ARID1, RHOA, and CDH1 mutations and fusions involving RHO-family GTPase-activating proteins. The integrated analysis showed elevated expression of cell adhesion and angiogenesis-related pathways.

Tumors with CIN are frequently located at the gastroesophageal junction or cardia and generally correspond to the intestinal type. These tumors show marked aneuploidy and highly variable chromosomal copy numbers, as well as frequent mutations of the tumor suppressor gene TP53. Additionally, amplifications including epidermal growth factor receptor (EGFR), ERBB2 (HER2), ERBB3, fibroblast growth factor receptor 2 (FGFR2), MET proto-oncogene (MET), vascular endothelial growth factor A (VEGFA), and KRAS/NRAS are frequent. Notably, some of these amplified RTKs may be blocked by targeted therapies that are currently used or under development.

The Asian Cancer Research Group (ACRG)

The ACRG evaluated 300 primary gastric cancer tumors (Cristescu 2015) and defined four molecular subtypes based on gene expression data: MSI (~23%), epithelial-mesenchymal-like (~15%), TP53 active (~26%), and TP53 inactive (~36%). These subtypes were associated with distinct genomic alterations, survival outcomes, and recurrence patterns after surgery.

Microsatellite-unstable tumors (MSI) are hypermutated tumors occurring in the antrum and showing intestinal histology. This subgroup was mostly diagnosed at an earlier stage and has the best overall prognosis and the lowest frequency of recurrence of the four subtypes. MLH1 expression is lost and can be detected by immunohistochemistry. This subtype was associated with hypermutation, including mutations in KRAS, ALK, ARID1A, and the PI3K-PTEN-mTOR pathway.

The mesenchymal-like type (MSS/EMT) corresponds to an epithelial to mesenchymal (EMT) gene expression signature, shows CDH1 expression loss, and exhibits diffuse histology. This subgroup preferentially occurs at an earlier age and shows the worst prognosis, is diagnosed mostly at an advanced stage and has the highest recurrence frequency of the four subtypes. These tumors showed a lower number of mutations than other MSS subtypes.

Non-MSI and non-EMT have intermediate prognosis and recurrence rates and were further divided into TP53 active (MSS/TP53+) and TP53 inactive (MSS/TP53-) using a two-gene (CDKN1A (p21) and MDM2) TP53-activity signature. The TP53-active subgroup showed a better prognosis and was enriched in EBV-positive cases. MSS/TP53+tumors showed the highest prevalence of TP53 mutations, while MSS/TP53- tumors showed a relatively higher frequency of mutations in APC, ARID1A, KRAS, PIK3CA, and SMAD4 compared to MSS/TP53+ subgroup.

Table 5. ACRG molecular classification

- MSI
  - Antrum
  - Intestinal histology
  - MLH1 expression loss
  - Hypermutation: KRAS, ALK, ARID1A, PI3K-PTEN-mTOR pathway
  - Overexpression of PDL1
- Mesenchymal-like (MSS/EMT)
  - Younger patients
  - Diffuse histology
- TP53 active (MSS/TP53+)
  - EBV-positive enriched
  - Mutations in APC, ARID1A, KRAS, PIK3CA, and SMAD4
- TP53 inactive (MSS/TP53-)
  - TP53 mutations

Clinical Relevance of Molecular Classifications

Molecular subtypes defined by the ACRG were associated in the initial classification report with survival outcome and recurrence patterns after surgery [19]. Although the TCGA classification did not initially show prognostic significance, later studies stratified patients by survival and adjuvant chemotherapy outcomes using this classification, with EBV subtype associated with the best prognosis, and GS subtype with the worst prognosis [18, 51]. This agrees with previous reports finding a better prognosis of EBV-positive tumors [52–54]. Although this association has not been consistently observed [41]. MSI high tumors, a subgroup recognized in both classifications, have also been related with a better outcome [55, 56].

In contrast to other cancer types, such as breast carcinoma, molecular classification of gastric cancer does not yet contribute to targeted therapies. However, both EBV positive tumors, which show frequent PD-L1 amplification, and MSI high tumors, highly hypermutated, are susceptible to treatment with immune checkpoint inhibitors. Notably, immunohistochemical evaluation of MMR proteins and in situ hybridization analysis of EBV are reliable and feasible methods, so that routine incorporation of these biomarkers may help to establish more personalized treatment regimes [7, 57–59]. The current American Joint Committee on Cancer (AJCC) staging manual recommends MSI testing in patients with gastric cancer [60]. According to the current WHO classification of gastrointestinal tumors, routine evaluation for MSI and PD-L1 expression is not recommended, although it is recognized that gastric adenocarcinomas are potential candidates for immunotherapy [3]. Patients with GC associated with MSI and EBV showed a remarkable response to pembrolizumab and high correlation with PD-L1 positivity [61-62].

References

[1] Smyth E, Verheij M, Allum W, Cunningham D, Cervantes A, Arnold D. ESMO Guidelines Committee. et al. Gastric cancer: ESMO clinical practice guidelines for diagnosis, treatment and follow-up. *Ann Oncol 2016;* 27, v38–v49.

[2] Rawla P, Barsouk A. Epidemiology of gastric cancer: Global trends, risk factors and prevention. *Prz. Gastroentero 2019;* 14, 26–38.

[3] Nagtegaal I, D Odze R, Klimstra D, Paradis V, Rugge M, Schirmacher P, Washington K, Carneiro F, Cree I, WHO Classification of Tumours Editorial Board. The 2019 WHO classification of tumours of the digestive system. *Histopathology 2020;* 76, 182–188.

[4] Plummer M, Franceschi S, Vignat J, Forman D, De Martel C. Global burden of gastric cancer attributable to pylori. *Int. J. Cancer 2015;* 136, 487–490 (2015).

[5] ASGE Standards of Practice Committee; Evans J, Chandrasekhara V, Chathadi K, Decker A, Early D, Fisher D, Foley K, Hwang J, Jue T, Lightdale J, Pasha S, Sharaf R, Shergill A, Cash B, DeWitt J. The role of endoscopy in the management of premalignant and malignant conditions of the stomach. *Gastrointest Endosc 2015;* 82, 1–8.

[6] Banks M, Graham D, Jansen J, Gotoda T, Coda S, di Pietro M, Uedo N, Bhandari P, Pritchard M, Kuipers E, Rodriguez-Justo M, Novelli M, Ragunath K, Shepherd N, Dinis-Ribeiro M. British Society of Gastroenterology guidelines on the diagnosis and management of patients at risk of gastric adenocarcinoma. *Gut 2019;* 68, 1545–1575.

[7] Martinez-Ciarpaglini C, Fleitas-Kanonnikoff T, Gambardella V, Llorca M, Mongort C, Mengual R, Nieto G, Navarro L, Huerta M, Rosello S, Roda D, Tarazona N, Navarro N, Ribas G, Cervantes A. Assessing molecular subtypes of gastric cancer: Microsatellite unstable and Epstein-Barr virus subtypes. Methods for detection and clinical and pathological implications. *ESMO Open 2019;* 4, 1–

[8] Mathiak M, Warneke VS, Behrens HM, Haag J, Böger C, Krüger S, Röcken C. Clinicopathologic Characteristics of Microsatellite

Instable Gastric Carcinomas Revisited: Urgent Need for Standardization. *Appl Immunohistochem Mol Morphol.* 2017;25(1):12-24.

[9] Dong J, Thrift AP. Alcohol, smoking and risk of oesophago-gastric cancer. *Best Pract. Res. Clin. Gastroenterol 2017.* 31, 509–517.

[10] Rota M, Pelucchi C, Bertuccio P, Matsuo K, Zhang ZF, Ito H, Hu J, Johnson KC, Palli D, Ferraroni M, Yu GP, Muscat J, Lunet N, Peleteiro B, Ye W, Song H, Zaridze D, Maximovitch D, Guevara M, Fernández-Villa T, Vioque J, Navarrete-Muñoz EM, Wolk A, Orsini N, Bellavia A, Håkansson N, Mu L, Persiani R, Kurtz RC, Lagiou A, Lagiou P, Galeone C, Bonzi R, Boffetta P, Boccia S, Negri E, La Vecchia C. Alcohol consumption and gastric cancer risk-A pooled analysis within the StoP project consortium. *Int J Cancer.* 2017;141(10):1950-1962.

[11] Lauren, P. the Two Histological Main Types of Gastric Carcinoma: Diffuse and So-Called Intestinal-Type Carcinoma. an Attempt At a Histo-Clinical Classification. *Acta Pathol Microbiol Scand. 1965;* 64, 31–49.

[12] Berlth F, Bollschweiler E, Drebber U, Hoelscher AH, Moenig S. Pathohistological classification systems in gastric cancer: diagnostic relevance and prognostic value. *World J Gastroenterol.* 2014;20(19):5679-5684.

[13] *WHO Classification of Tumours of the Digestive System.*

[14] Nakamura K, Sugano H, Takagi K. Carcinoma of the stomach in incipient phase: its histogenesis and histological appearances. *Gan.* 1968;59(3):251-8.

[15] Mulligan R, Rember R. Histogenesis and biologic behavior of gastric carcinoma: study of one hundred thirty-eight cases. *AMA Arch Pathol.* 1954;58(1):1-25.

[16] Goseki N, Takizawa T, Koike M. Differences in the mode of the extension of gastric cancer classified by histological type: new histological classification of gastric carcinoma. *Gut.* 1992;33(5):606-12.

[17] Carneiro F. Classification of gastric carcinomas. *Current Diagnostic Pathology, 1997; 4(1)51-59.*

[18] Cancer Genome Atlas Research Network. Comprehensive molecular characterization of gastric adenocarcinoma. *Nature.* 2014;513(7517):202-209.

[19] Cristescu R, Lee J, Nebozhyn M, Kim KM, Ting JC, Wong SS, Liu J, Yue YG, Wang J, Yu K, Ye XS, Do IG, Liu S, Gong L, Fu J, Jin JG, Choi MG, Sohn TS, Lee JH, Bae JM, Kim ST, Park SH, Sohn I, Jung SH, Tan P, Chen R, Hardwick J, Kang WK, Ayers M, Hongyue D, Reinhard C, Loboda A, Kim S, Aggarwal A. Molecular analysis of gastric cancer identifies subtypes associated with distinct clinical outcomes. *Nat Med.* 2015;21(5):449-56.

[20] Ikoma N, Agnes A, Chen HC, Wang X, Blum MM, Das P, Minsky B, Estrella JS, Mansfield P, Ajani JA, Badgwell BD. Linitis Plastica: a Distinct Type of Gastric Cancer. *J Gastrointest Surg.* 2020;24(5):1018-1025.

[21] Shah MA, Khanin R, Tang L, Janjigian YY, Klimstra DS, Gerdes H, Kelsen DP. Molecular classification of gastric cancer: a new paradigm. *Clin Cancer Res.* 2011;17(9):2693-701.

[22] Chen YC, Fang WL, Wang RF, Liu CA, Yang MH, Lo SS, Wu CW, Li AF, Shyr YM, Huang KH. Clinicopathological Variation of Lauren Classification in Gastric Cancer. *Pathol Oncol Res.* 2016;22 (1):197-202.

[23] Japanese Gastric Cancer Association. Japanese classification of gastric carcinoma: 3rd English edition. *Gastric Cancer.* 2011; 14(2):101-12.

[24] Jiménez-Fonseca P, Carmona-Bayonas A, Hernández R, Custodio A, Cano JM, Lacalle A, Echavarria I, Macias I, Mangas M, Visa L, Buxo E, Álvarez Manceñido F, Viudez A, Pericay C, Azkarate A, Ramchandani A, López C, Martinez de Castro E, Fernández Montes A, Longo F, Sánchez Bayona R, Limón ML, Diaz-Serrano A, Martin Carnicero A, Arias D, Cerdà P, Rivera F, Vieitez JM, Sánchez Cánovas M, Garrido M, Gallego J. Lauren subtypes of advanced gastric cancer influence survival and response to chemotherapy: real-

world data from the AGAMENON National Cancer Registry. *Br J Cancer*. 2017;117(6):775-782.

[25] Yu CC, Levison DA, Dunn JA, Ward LC, Demonakou M, Allum WH, Hallisey MT. Pathological prognostic factors in the second British Stomach Cancer Group trial of adjuvant therapy in resectable gastric cancer. *Br J Cancer*. 1995;71(5):1106-10.

[26] Luu C, Thapa R, Woo K, Coppola D, Almhanna K, Pimiento JM, Chen DT, Marquez DD, Hodul PJ. Does histology really influence gastric cancer prognosis? *J Gastrointest Oncol*. 2017;8(6):1026-1036.

[27] Mönig S, Baldus SE, Collet PH, Zirbes TK, Bollschweiler E, Thiele J, Dienes HP, Hölscher AH. Histological grading in gastric cancer by Goseki classification: correlation with histopathological subtypes and prognosis. *Anticancer Res*. 2001;21:617-20.

[28] Zhao LY, Wang JJ, Zhao YL, Chen XZ, Yang K, Chen XL, Zhang WH, Liu K, Song XH, Zheng JB, Zhou ZG, Yu PW, Li Y, Hu JK. Superiority of Tumor Location-Modified Lauren Classification System for Gastric Cancer: A Multi-Institutional Validation Analysis. *Ann Surg Oncol*. 2018;25(11):3257-3263.

[29] Song Z, Wu Y, Yang J, Yang D, Fang X. Progress in the treatment of advanced gastric cancer. *Tumour Biol*. 2017;39(7):101042 8317714626.

[30] Asplund J, Kauppila JH, Mattsson F, Lagergren J. Survival Trends in Gastric Adenocarcinoma: A Population-Based Study in Sweden. *Ann Surg Oncol*. 2018;25(9):2693-2702.

[31] Kim KJ, Lee TH, Cho NY, Yang HK, Kim WH, Kang GH. Differential clinicopathologic features in microsatellite-unstable gastric cancers with and without MLH1 methylation. *Hum Pathol*. 2013;44(6):1055-64.

[32] Mariette C, Carneiro F, Grabsch HI, van der Post RS, Allum W, de Manzoni G; European Chapter of International Gastric Cancer Association. Consensus on the pathological definition and classification of poorly cohesive gastric carcinoma. *Gastric Cancer*. 2019;22(1):1-9.

[33] Gong YB, Zhu Z, Wang X, Xu HM. [Influence of different biological behaviors on prognosis of patients with advanced gastric cancer at the same TNM stage]. *Zhonghua Wei Chang Wai Ke Za Zhi.* 2020;23(10):953-962.

[34] Wong HH, Chu P. Immunohistochemical features of the gastrointestinal tract tumors. *J Gastrointest Oncol.* 2012;3(3):262-84.

[35] O'Connell FP, Wang HH, Odze RD. Utility of immunohistochemistry in distinguishing primary adenocarcinomas from metastatic breast carcinomas in the gastrointestinal tract. *Arch Pathol Lab Med.* 2005;129(3):338-47.

[36] A Pereira MA, Ramos MFKP, Faraj SF, Dias AR, Yagi OK, Zilberstein B, Cecconello I, Alves VAF, de Mello ES, Ribeiro U Jr. Clinicopathological and prognostic features of Epstein-Barr virus infection, microsatellite instability, and PD-L1 expression in gastric cancer. *J Surg Oncol.* 2018;117(5):829-839.

[37] Boland CR, Thibodeau SN, Hamilton SR, Sidransky D, Eshleman JR, Burt RW, Meltzer SJ, Rodriguez-Bigas MA, Fodde R, Ranzani GN, Srivastava S. A National Cancer Institute Workshop on Microsatellite Instability for cancer detection and familial predisposition: development of international criteria for the determination of microsatellite instability in colorectal cancer. *Cancer Res.* 1998;58(22):5248-57.

[38] Umar A, Boland CR, Terdiman JP, Syngal S, de la Chapelle A, Rüschoff J, Fishel R, Lindor NM, Burgart LJ, Hamelin R, Hamilton SR, Hiatt RA, Jass J, Lindblom A, Lynch HT, Peltomaki P, Ramsey SD, Rodriguez-Bigas MA, Vasen HF, Hawk ET, Barrett JC, Freedman AN, Srivastava S. Revised Bethesda Guidelines for hereditary nonpolyposis colorectal cancer (Lynch syndrome) and microsatellite instability. *J Natl Cancer Inst.* 2004;96(4):261-8.

[39] Grogg KL, Lohse CM, Pankratz VS, Halling KC, Smyrk TC. Lymphocyte-rich gastric cancer: associations with Epstein-Barr virus, microsatellite instability, histology, and survival. *Mod Pathol*;16(7):641-51.

[40] Hissong E, Ramrattan G, Zhang P, Zhou XK, Young G, Klimstra DS, Shia J, Fernandes H, Yantiss RK. Gastric Carcinomas With Lymphoid Stroma: An Evaluation of the Histopathologic and Molecular Features. *Am J Surg Pathol*;42(4):453-462.

[41] Kijima Y, Ishigami S, Hokita S, Koriyama C, Akiba S, Eizuru Y, Aikou T. The comparison of the prognosis between Epstein-Barr virus (EBV)-positive gastric carcinomas and EBV-negative ones. *Cancer Lett.* 2003;200(1):33-40.

[42] Herath CH, Chetty R. Epstein-Barr virus-associated lymphoepithelioma-like gastric carcinoma. *Arch Pathol Lab Med.* 2008;132(4):706-9.

[43] Kim GH, Ahn JY, Jung HY, Park YS, Kim MJ, Choi KD, Lee JH, Choi KS, Kim DH, Lim H, Song HJ, Lee GH, Kim JH. Clinical and Endoscopic Features of Metastatic Tumors in the Stomach. *Gut* Liver. 2015;9(5):615-22.

[44] Almubarak MM, Laé M, Cacheux W, de Cremoux P, Pierga JY, Reyal F, Bennett SP, Falcou MC, Salmon RJ, Baranger B, Mariani P. Gastric metastasis of breast cancer: a single centre retrospective study. *Dig Liver Dis.* 2011;43(10):823-7.

[45] Geada L, Kantor M, Mohan K, Weingrad D, Nasiff LS. An Uncommon Presentation of a Common Disease: A Review of Gastric Metastasis From Breast Carcinoma. *Cureus.* 2020;12(12):e11920.

[46] Miettinen M, McCue PA, Sarlomo-Rikala M, Rys J, Czapiewski P, Wazny K, Langfort R, Waloszczyk P, Biernat W, Lasota J, Wang Z. GATA3: a multispecific but potentially useful marker in surgical pathology: a systematic analysis of 2500 epithelial and nonepithelial tumors. *Am J Surg Pathol.* 2014;38(1):13-22.

[47] Song W, Liu F, Wang S, Shi H, He W, He Y. Primary gastric malignant melanoma: challenge in preoperative diagnosis. *Int J Clin Exp Pathol.* 2014;7(10):6826-31.

[48] Mellotte GS, Sabu D, O'Reilly M, McDermott R, O'Connor A, Ryan BM. The challenge of primary gastric melanoma: a systematic review. *Melanoma Manag.* 2020;7(4):MMT51.

[49] Mohamed A, Gonzalez RS, Lawson D, Wang J, Cohen C. SOX10 expression in malignant melanoma, carcinoma, and normal tissues. *Appl Immunohistochem Mol Morphol*. 2013;21(6):506-10.

[50] Ratti M, Lampis A, Hahne JC, Passalacqua R, Valeri N. Microsatellite instability in gastric cancer: molecular bases, clinical perspectives, and new treatment approaches. *Cell Mol Life Sci*. 2018;75(22):4151-4162.

[51] Sohn BH, Hwang JE, Jang HJ, Lee HS, Oh SC, Shim JJ, Lee KW, Kim EH, Yim SY, Lee SH, Cheong JH, Jeong W, Cho JY, Kim J, Chae J, Lee J, Kang WK, Kim S, Noh SH, Ajani JA, Lee JS. Clinical Significance of Four Molecular Subtypes of Gastric Cancer Identified by The Cancer Genome Atlas Project. *Clin Cancer Res*. 2017; 26:10.1158/1078-0432.CCR-16-2211.

[52] Van Beek J, zur Hausen A, Klein Kranenbarg E, van de Velde CJ, Middeldorp JM, van den Brule AJ, Meijer CJ, Bloemena E. EBV-positive gastric adenocarcinomas: a distinct clinicopathologic entity with a low frequency of lymph node involvement. *J Clin Oncol*. 2004;22(4):664-70.

[53] Camargo MC, Kim WH, Chiaravalli AM, Kim KM, Corvalan AH, Matsuo K, Yu J, Sung JJ, Herrera-Goepfert R, Meneses-Gonzalez F, Kijima Y, Natsugoe S, Liao LM, Lissowska J, Kim S, Hu N, Gonzalez CA, Yatabe Y, Koriyama C, Hewitt SM, Akiba S, Gulley ML, Taylor PR, Rabkin CS. Improved survival of gastric cancer with tumour Epstein-Barr virus positivity: an international pooled analysis. *Gut*;63(2):236-43.

[54] Yi M, Jiao D, Xu H, Liu Q, Zhao W, Han X, Wu K. Biomarkers for predicting efficacy of PD-1/PD-L1 inhibitors. *Mol Cancer*. 2018;17(1):129.

[55] Marrelli D, Polom K, Pascale V, Vindigni C, Piagnerelli R, De Franco L, Ferrara F, Roviello G, Garosi L, Petrioli R, Roviello F. Strong Prognostic Value of Microsatellite Instability in Intestinal Type Non-cardia Gastric Cancer. *Ann Surg Oncol*. 2016;23(3):943-50.

[56] Zhu L, Li Z, Wang Y, Zhang C, Liu Y, Qu X. Microsatellite instability and survival in gastric cancer: A systematic review and meta-analysis. *Mol Clin Oncol.* 2015;3(3):699-705.

[57] Y Yoon JY, Sy K, Brezden-Masley C, Streutker CJ. Histo- and immunohistochemistry-based estimation of the TCGA and ACRG molecular subtypes for gastric carcinoma and their prognostic significance: A single-institution study. *PLoS One.* 2019;14(12):e0224812.

[58] Luchini C, Bibeau F, Ligtenberg MJL, Singh N, Nottegar A, Bosse T, Miller R, Riaz N, Douillard JY, Andre F, Scarpa A. ESMO recommendations on microsatellite instability testing for immunotherapy in cancer, and its relationship with PD-1/PD-L1 expression and tumour mutational burden: a systematic review-based approach. *Ann Oncol.* 2019;30(8):1232-1243. doi:

[59] Birkman EM, Mansuri N, Kurki S, Ålgars A, Lintunen M, Ristamäki R, Sundström J, Carpén O. Gastric cancer: immunohistochemical classification of molecular subtypes and their association with clinicopathological characteristics. *Virchows Arch.* 2018;472(3):369-382.

[60] Amin, M. B., Edge, S. B. & American Joint Committee on Cancer. *AJCC cancer staging manual*. (2017).

[61] Kim ST, Cristescu R, Bass AJ, Kim KM, Odegaard JI, Kim K, Liu XQ, Sher X, Jung H, Lee M, Lee S, Park SH, Park JO, Park YS, Lim HY, Lee H, Choi M, Talasaz A, Kang PS, Cheng J, Loboda A, Lee J, Kang WK. Comprehensive molecular characterization of clinical responses to PD-1 inhibition in metastatic gastric cancer. *Nat Med.* 2018;24(9):1449-1458.

[62] Smyth EC, Wotherspoon A, Peckitt C, Gonzalez D, Hulkki-Wilson S, Eltahir Z, Fassan M, Rugge M, Valeri N, Okines A, Hewish M, Allum W, Stenning S, Nankivell M, Langley R, Cunningham D. Mismatch Repair Deficiency, Microsatellite Instability, and Survival: An Exploratory Analysis of the Medical Research Council Adjuvant Gastric Infusional Chemotherapy (MAGIC) Trial. *JAMA Oncol.* 2017;3(9):1197-1203.

In: Gastric Peritoneal Carcinomatosis ISBN: 978-1-53619-487-6
Editors: F. López Mozos et al.

Chapter 5

PATIENT SELECTION AND PREOPERATIVE CONSIDERATIONS

M. E. Barrios*, MD, M. C. Fernández, MD and R. Martí Fernández, MD
Hospital Clínico Universitario,
Valencia, Spain

ABSTRACT

Introduction

The presence of peritoneal carcinomatosis (PC) in a patient affected from gastric cancer is associated to a dim prognosis and the median survival of these patients with systemic chemotherapy is approximately 6.7 months. To determine which group of patients would benefit from an aggressive treatment course such as cytorreductive surgery (CRS) and hypertermic intraperitoneal chemotherapy (HIPEC) strict selection criteria and different measures have been employed to assure patients would endure the procedure and also arise from it with an acceptable quality of life.

---

* Corresponding author's E-mail: barriosmariu@gmail.com.

Patient Selection

Elderly patients (generally over 70 years old) with major comorbidities or patients with poor performance status (ECOG > 2) have been commonly excluded from this procedure. Patients susceptible of eligibility for CRS must be evaluated with CT scans or PET CT to rule out distant metastases and preoperatively estimate PCI in an attempt to identify radiological findings that might indicate or predict impossibility to achieve complete resections.

Preoperative Considerations

The procedure of CRS and HIPEC is long and bears great risk of major morbidity and mortality. The aim of preoperative assessment is to determine as accurate as possible a patient´s physical and medical condition, the ability to tolerate the surgical procedure and anaesthesia.

Prehabilitation includes nutritional assessment and support; abstinence from smoking/alcohol and other addictions as well as physical and psychological optimization.

High morbidity rates of CRS and the short median survival associated to gastric cancer PC have driven surgeons to attempt to narrow the inclusion criteria for it, and once proven eligible, to improve patient´s preoperative state to up their chances of emerging from it with good results; consequently resorting to prehabilitation protocols.

Conclusion

The effectiveness of prehabilitation regimes has been demonstrated in a variety of scenarios including gynecologic, cardiothoracic, general surgery (colonic, bariatric, etc.) and orthopedic. This wide range of procedures and patients characteristics seem to prove that prehabilitiation programs could be tailored to different types of patients and disease related specific morbidity, hence the idea to implement this concept to cytorreductive surgery.

Introduction

The presence of peritoneal carcinomatosis (PC) in a patient affected from gastric cancer is associated with a dim prognosis as with most of the solid tumors that can originate it.

The median survival of these patients albeit poor can be prolonged with systemic chemotherapy approximately 6.7 months more than best supportive care [1].

Cytorreductive surgery (CRS) and hypertermic intraperitoneal chemotherapy (HIPEC) emerged as an interesting weapon to manage peritoneal metastases. Some studies have suggested it could become curative treatment in a select group of patients with low volume peritoneal disease [2]. With this similar premise in mind Rihuete found and increased median survival of 19 months for patients with peritoneal carcinomatosis from gastric cancer treated with CRS and HIPEC (PCI < 6) [3].

To better determine which group of patients would benefit from this aggressive treatment course strict selection criteria and different measures have been employed to assure patients would not only endure the procedure but arise from it with an acceptable quality of life.

Patient Selection

The successful treatment of PC amongst other things requires proper patient selection. To achieve this, surgeons must take into considerations different factors and characteristics of the patients, the tumor itself and extent of peritoneal involvement.

Elderly patients (generally over 70 years old) with major comorbidities or patients with poor performance status (ECOG > 2) have been commonly excluded from this procedure given its aggressive nature and their presumed frailty to withstand it. Regarding the extent of the disease: Mesenteric root infiltration, small bowel resection exceeding more than one-third of the whole length of the bowel, massive retroperitoneal involvement, massively infiltrated pancreatic capsule, and unresectable liver metastases (more than 3 liver metastases or metastases that require major liver resections) are generally accepted absolute exclusion criteria for radical CRS regardless of the PC origin [4].

Grade	ECOG
0	Fully active, able to carry on all predisease performance without restriction
1	Restricted in physically strenuous activity but ambulatory and able to carry out work of a light or sedentary nature—for example, light house work, office work
2	Ambulatory and capable of all self-care but unable to carry out any work activities. Up and about more than 50% of waking hours
3	Capable of only limited self-care, confined to bed or chair more than 50% of waking hours
4	Completely disabled. Cannot carry on any self-care. Totally confined to bed or chair
5	Dead

ECOG, Eastern Cooperative Oncology Group.

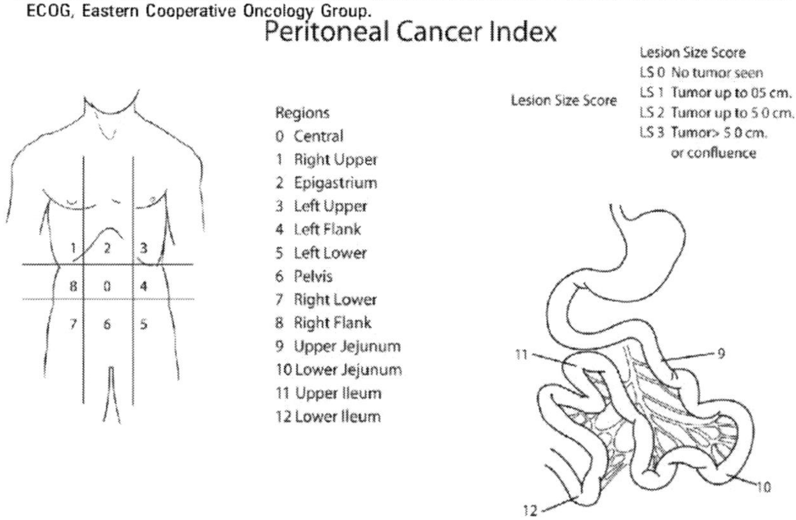

Figure 1. Sugarbaker peritoneal carcinomatosis index PCI.

The peritoneal carcinomatosis index (PCI) is useful to assess the degree of peritoneal spread, and for both operability and prognosis [8]. This classification system divides the abdomen into 9 sectors and the small bowel into 4 more sectors. The total score is calculated according to lesion size scores of each sector with a maximum score of 39 (Figure 1) [9].

When determined preoperatively through imaging techniques it must be taken into consideration that radiologic PCI often underestimates the actual amount of peritoneal disease (difficult to evaluate compromised bowel or to see small volume lesions with CT showing a sensitivity ranging from 8 - 17%) [10]. On this preoperative setting PCI can be helpful to plan the surgical strategy or decide whether or not to perform the procedure but it is most accurately described intraoperatively. CRS and HIPEC for peritoneal carcinomatosis from gastric cancer should be considered in selected patients when the surgeon is confident that a CC0 (Table 1) is possible to obtain [15].

A metanalysis by Desiderio [11] found no statistically significant differences in survival rates when analyzed by the extent of carcinomatosis between the limited peritoneal dissemination and extensive peritoneal dissemination groups. Similar to the findings of Yang [5] when compared low PCI (<20) and high PCI (> 20).

Table 1. The Completeness of Cytorreduction Score

SCORE	DEFINITION
CC-0	No residual tumor seen
CC-1	Residual tumor nodules <2.5mm
CC-2	Residual tumor nodules ≥2.5mm ≤2.5cm
CC-3	Residual tumor nodules ≥2.5cm

Other studies have found differences in patients with lower PCI or to be more specific lower than 15 [3, 12-14, 26-27]. In this particular group of patients CRS + HIPEC has shown an overall survival above 12 months, and can go as high as 18 months for those with PCI lower than 6 [12-13].

Hotopp found that overall survival significantly worsened after the resection of more than 5 organs and therefore assumed that higher PCI could correlate to the extent of resection and poor prognosis associated to PCI > 12 [25]. Rudloff et al. set the limit for a PCI of ≤15 [26], while Glehen et al. questioned the usefulness of the surgical procedure from a PCI of 12 [27].

A prospective randomized trial demonstrated that CRS and HIPEC provides survival benefit with a median overall survival (OS) of 11 months for patients with synchronous PC from gastric cancer when compared with 6 months OS when patients were offered CRS alone [5].

These results displayed a difference in OS relating to the onset of PC, with metacronous disease showing a worse prognosis similarly to the results found by Glehen [6]. Since PC is difficult to detect through standard imaging techniques this makes it challenging to diagnose metachronous disease in time to consired it resectable, this could be the reason why some surgeons consider sinchronous PC to be more treatable than metachronous PC [15].

The subgroup analysis of the German database study found that patients with incomplete cytoreduction or PCI > 15 would not benefit form CRS + HIPEC based on an overall survival of 10 or 5 months respectively. We could say based on this and other results that CRS including gastrectomy in patients with a PCI > 12 should not be recommended [12, 14].

Additionally, numerous phase III randomized trials being conducted across the world are attempting to better determine the selection criteria for CRS/HIPEC [7].

Preoperative Considerations

The procedure of CRS and HIPEC is generally long and bears great risk of major morbidity and mortality. Complications of this intervention are related to the extent of peritonectomies and resections, number of anastomoses, duration of the surgery and doses of cytotoxic chemotherapeutic drugs used in HIPEC [4].

CRS and HIPEC for PC of gastric cancer has similar morbidity and mortality rates when compared with PC of other origins [15] this could be due to patients status at the time of performing the surgery. Patients with PC usually suffer malnourishment, important psychological distress and physical morbidity related both to the disease and to the impact of previously received treatments.

These patients could benefit from prehabilitation or enhanced recovery protocols to improve their quality of life after surgery. Enhanced recovery after surgery (ERAS) protocols were first applied and demonstrated their validity on patients with colonic resection.

On these patients the adoption of ERAS pathways with a high compliance showed significant reduction of postoperative complications, length of hospital stay and costs.

Lu et al. demonstrated that for patients undergoing CRS and HIPEC the implementation of prehabilitation in an enhanced recovery after surgery protocol was associated with decreased hospital length of stay and days hospitalized in an intensive care unit without increasing postoperative complications or unplanned 30-d readmission [24]. Although this study was not specific for PC of gastric cancer (most of the patients had other origins for PC), the premises they discovered could still apply to gastric cancer PC since the basis of CRS are the same to all PC regardless of their origin.

Efforts have been made to assess and standardize ERAS protocols for cytorreductive surgery disregarding the origin of PC [16, 18]. These protocols entail measures to be performed in different periods including preoperative, intraoperative and postoperative.

The aim of preoperative assessment is to determine as accurate as possible a patient´s physical and medical condition, the ability to tolerate the surgical procedure and anaesthesia. Prehabilitation includes nutritional assessment and support; abstinence from smoking/alcohol and other addictions as well as physical and psychological optimization. Systemic chemotherapy, if ongoing, should be interrupted at least 6 weeks prior to surgery [17].

Preoperative Information and Psychological Counselling

At the first visit the surgeon has the opportunity to discuss different treatment courses and options with special consideration owing to the fact that making the decision to proceed with CRS and HIPEC can be challenging for both patient and surgeon.

This is also the opportunity to introduce the principles of prehabilitation to the patient knowing that all this information can arouse fears about surgery, postoperative results and expectations. Written and online information are useful resources to inform and help reassure patients and their families.

ERAS protocols for major abdominal procedures recommend pre-operative counselling to decrease anxiety, improve pain management and increase patient satisfaction.

A review suggested that psychological counselling before surgery potentially improves quality of life, somatic symptoms and psychological outcomes reported by the patients [18].

Nutritional Assessment and Optimization

Accurately determining a patient´s nutritional status is one of the most important steps of prehabilitation. There are several nutritional scores that could be employed such as the MUST (Malnutrition Universal Screening Tool), the SNAQ (Short Nutritional Assessment Questionnaire) and the PONS (PreOperative Nutrition Score) which is a modification of MUST tool that includes serum albumin levels to help determine nutritional status and risk of postoperative complications.

For patients with low nutritional risk calculated by means of one of the aforementioned scales, a high protein diet is indicated with at least 1.2 – 2.0g protein/kg per day since 1 week prior to and 1 week after the surgery. Immunomodulatory supplements 3 times a day after surgery are also permitted. Patients with or at risk for malnutrition, supplementation (oral>enteral>parenteral) of nutrients and protein (>1.2g/kg/day) as well as oral nutritional supplements for at least 5 days and up to 14 days (in cases of severe malnutrition) prior to surgery should be indicated routinely. Oral immunonutrition for 5/7 days before the surgical procedure might help reduce postoperative (infectious) complications. Some patients may require hospitalization for enteral (tube feeding) or parenteral nutrition in case of severe malnutrition.

Cessation of Smoking and Alcohol Consumption

Cigarette smoking and moderate to heavy alcohol consumption are associated with cardiovascular disease and wound related complications. Moreover, alcohol has also been identified as cause for a weakened immune system, bleeding complications and delayed recovery.

In the United States of America a "Standard Drink" has been defined by The National Institute on Alcohol Abuse and Alcoholism (NIAAA) as 14 grams of pure alcohol. "At-risk" or "heavy drinking" is defined as 4 drinks on any day for men and 3 drinks per day for women or 14 drinks per week for men and 7 per week for women. Patients identified as heavy alcohol consumers should be submitted to an intensive alcohol cessation program, including pharmacological intervention if necessary at least four weeks before surgery.

On the other hand, smoking is an entire risk factor in itself and has been linked to increased postoperative morbidity including but not limited to pulmonary complications, infections and higher rates of admission to intensive care units. Since the best timing for smoking cessation is unknown, patients should be advised to stop smoking as soon as possible. Intensive behavioral changes and nicotine replacement, at least four weeks ahead of surgery must be advised and indicated routinely.

Hematologic Support and Physical Exercise

Anemia is a common result on the preoperative work up of oncologic patients and has a wide variety of causes (iron, folate or vitamin B12 deficiency or chronic renal insufficiency), this finding is associated with adverse outcomes including cardiac events and death [19]. Patients planned for major abdominal surgery should be tested for anemia at least 30 days before the procedure to allow enough time for correction.

Immediate medical therapy (oral/intravenous iron, folate/vitamin B12 or erythropoietin treatment) could be prescribed and preoperative transfusions are reserved for severe refractory situations preferably except in cases of haemoglobinopathies such as sickle cell disease.

A patient´s physical condition is also of the outmost importance to the recovery process, the recommended test to accurately determine this condition include: "Six-minute walk test" with control of cardiac frequency and oxygen saturation and shallow assessment of respiratory status (respiratory pattern, thoracometry, modified MRI and Borg dyspnea scale). Currently, there are no specific guidelines for exercise neither resistance nor cardiovascular that could apply to the prehabilitation period.

The American Cancer Society guidelines suggest a minimum of 150 minutes of moderate exercise per week or 75 minutes of high intensity if the patient can tolerate it, combined with 2 or 3 sessions of resistance exercises [20]. Training with an inspirometer before the surgical procedure to learn the breathing exercises and objectives for the postoperative period might be of help since after surgery patients should start using an inspirometer and mobilize early ideally on the first postoperative day. Other activities such as using a pedal exerciser, sitting on a chair and walking according to a scheduled routine help maintain body muscle mass and reduces the risk of deep venous thrombosis thus preventing pulmonary thromboembolism.

Anesthetic Assessment

Preferably, an anaesthesiologist specialized in CRS and HIPEC procedures should evaluate the patient before surgery, since the changes associated with this long and complex procedure might induce major organ dysfunction a detailed and thorough preoperative work up becomes crucial.

Patients with a history of heart disease or cardiotoxicity from previously received chemotherapy agents may need echocardiogram and stress testing as part of their preoperative evaluation. The rest of the general checkup consist of laboratory tests (complete blood count, metabolic including renal function and coagulation).

Also, screening for obstructive sleep apnea is advised to anticipate a need for respiratory support in the perioperative setting such as continuous positive airway pressure (CPAP). This visit with the anesthesiologist might be perfect time to explain to the patient the need for regional anesthesia (epidural), review patient´s current medication (stop anticoagulant or antiplatelet therapies) and start preoperative multimodal analgesia to help reduce postoperative opioid consumption and restore bowel function.

Bowel Preparation

Cytorreductive procedures often include multiple bowel resections, anastomoses and pelvic en-bloc resections, this raises the question of mechanical bowel preparation (MBP) with or without oral antibiotics (OAB) or the latter alone. MBP was used historically under the premise that it would decrease anastomotic leaks and surgical site infection, however multiple studies have failed to show this association. A recent meta-analysis reported that the use of MBP had no preventive effect on surgical site infection, anastomotic leak or reoperation rates [21]. Thus, OAB were also studied with the same interest as MBP and found that it could decrease surgical site infection at the expense of an increased risk of Clostridium difficile related morbidity [28].

On 2019, MBP + OAB was compared to no preoperative bowel preparation in the MOBILE trial, again no difference was found o surgical site infection, anastomotic dehiscence or reoperation rate between arms [22]. To this date a standard recommendation on preoperative bowel preparation has not been issued and several randomized controlled trials are attempting to answer this question, it seems that for patients undergoing CRS and HIPEC with a high probability of rectal resection preoperative bowel preparation with a combination of OAB and MBP could be indicated.

Fasting

Long periods of fasting over 8 hours before any major surgical procedure were generally accepted to prevent the risk of pulmonary aspirations associated to a full stomach. At present anaesthesia societies recommend short preoperative fasting of up to 6h for solids and 2h for liquids before surgery [23].

Conclusion

The success of any surgery relies amongst other things in a proper indication, to achieve this, surgeons must take into consideration many factors that could be summarized in careful and strict patient selection.

Cytorreductive surgery being a long and complex procedure that often requires multivisceral resections plus the added morbidity related to HIPEC and the pathophysiological response it triggers, makes patient selection all the more crucial for it.

Stablishing a cut of value for PCI to help select patients that would benefit from surgery has proven difficult, with different studies suggesting that patients whose PCI was lower than 12 would show greater benefits in survival. It could be assumed that a higher PCI would mean larger extent of resection, add morbidity, difficult probabilities of obtaining CC0 and therefore explain poor prognosis associated to PCI > 12.

High morbidity rates of CRS and the short median survival associated to gastric cancer PC have driven surgeons to attempt to narrow the inclusion criteria for it, and once proven eligible, to improve patient´s preoperative state to up their chances of emerging from it with good results and quality of life; consequently resorting to prehabilitation protocols.

The effectiveness of prehabilitation regimes has been demonstrated in a variety of scenarios including gynecologic, cardiothoracic, general surgery (colonic, bariatric, etc.) and orthopedic. This wide range of procedures and patients characteristics seem to prove that prehabilitiation programs could be tailored to different types of patients and disease related specific morbidity, hence the idea to implement this concept to cytorreductive surgery.

REFERENCES

[1] Wagner, A. D., Syn, N. L., Moehler, M., Grothe, W., Yong, W. P., Tai, B.-C. et al. Chemotherapy for advanced gastric cancer. *Cochrane Database Syst. Rev.*, 2017; 29:CD004064.

[2] Morales-Soriano, R., Esteve-Pérez, N., Segura-Sampedro, J. J., Cascales-Campos, P., Barrios, P. Spanish Group of Peritoneal Malignancy Surface (GECOP). Current practice in cytoreductive surgery and HIPEC for metastatic peritoneal disease: Spanish multicentric survey. *Eur. J. Surg. Oncol.,* 2018; 44:228 - 36.

[3] Rihuete Caro, C., Manzanedo, I., Pereira, F., Carrion-Alvarez, L., Serrano, Á., Pérez-Viejo, E. Cytoreductive surgery combined with hyperthermic intraperitoneal chemotherapy (HIPEC) in patients with gastric cancer and peritoneal carcinomatosis. *Eur. J. Surg. Oncol.,* 2018; 44:1805 - 10.

[4] Valle, M., Federici, O., Garofalo, A. Patient selection for cytoreductive surgery and hyperthermic intraperitoneal

chemotherapy, and role of laparoscopy in diagnosis, staging, and treatment. *Surg. Oncol. Clin. N Am.,* 2012; 21: 515 - 531.

[5] Yang, X.-J., Huang, C.-Q., Suo, T., Mei, L.-J., Yang, G.-L., Cheng, F.-L., Zhou, Y.-F., Xiong, B., Yonemura, Y. and Li, Y. Cytoreductive Surgery and Hyperthermic Intraperitoneal Chemotherapy Improves Survival of Patients with Peritoneal Carcinomatosis from Gastric Cancer: Final Results of a Phase III Randomized Clinical Trial. *Ann. Surg. Oncol.,* (2011) 18:1575 - 1581.

[6] Glehen, O., Schreiber, V., Cotte, E. et al. Cytoreductive surgery and intraperitoneal chemohyperthermia for peritoneal carcinomatosis arising from gastric cancer. *Arch. Surg.,* 2004; 139:20 - 6.

[7] Ji, Z.-H., Peng, K.-W., Yu, Y., Li, X.-B., Yonemura, Y., Liu, Y. et al. Current status and future prospects of clinical trials on CRS + HIPEC for gastric cancer peritoneal metastases. *Int. J. Hyperth.,* 2017; 33:562 - 70.

[8] Terzi, C., Arslan, N. C., Canda, A. E. Peritoneal carcinomatosis of gastrointestinal tumors: where are we now? *World J. Gastroenterol.,* 2014 Oct. 21; 20(39):14371 - 80.

[9] Sugarbaker, P. H. Surgical responsibilities in the management of peritoneal carcinomatosis. *J. Surg. Oncol.,* 2010; 101: 713 - 724.

[10] Montori, G., Coccolini, F., Ceresoli, M., Catena, F., Colaianni, N., Poletti, E. and Ansaloni, L. The Treatment of Peritoneal Carcinomatosis in Advanced Gastric Cancer: State of the Art. *Int. J. Surg. Oncol.,* 2014; 2014:912418.

[11] Desiderio, J., Chao, J., Melstrom, L., Warner, S., Tozzi, F., Fong, Y., Parisi, A. and Woo, Y. The Thirty-Year Experience - A Meta-analysis of Randomized and High Quality Non-Randomized Studies of Hyperthermic Intraperitoneal Chemotherapy (HIPEC) in the Treatment of Gastric Cancer. *Eur. J. Cancer,* 2017; 79: 1 - 14.

[12] Rau, B., Brandl, A., Piso, P., Pelz, J., Busch, P., Demtröder, C., Schüle, S., Schlitt, H. J., Roitman, M., Tepel, J., Sulkowski, U., Uzunoglu, F., Hünerbein, M., Hörbelt, R., Ströhlein, M., Beckert, S., Königsrainer, I., Königsrainer, A. Peritoneum Surface Oncology

Group and members of the StuDoQ|Peritoneum Registry of the German Society for General and Visceral Surgery (DGAV). Peritoneal metastasis in gastric cancer: results from the German database. *Gastric Cancer,* 2020 Jan.; 23(1):11 - 22.

[13] Manzanedo, I., Pereira, F., Rihuete, Caro, C., Pérez-Viejo, E., Serrano, Á., Gutiérrez Calvo, A., Regueira, F. M., Casado-Adam, Á., Cascales-Campos, P. A., Arteaga, X., García-Fadrique, A., Gómez Sanz, R., López García, A., Zozaya, G., Arjona, Á., Gil Martínez, J. Cytoreductive Surgery and Hyperthermic Intraperitoneal Chemotherapy (HIPEC) for Gastric Cancer with Peritoneal Carcinomatosis: Multicenter Study of Spanish Group of Peritoneal Oncologic Surgery (GECOP). *Ann. Surg. Oncol.,* 2019 Aug.; 26(8):2615 - 2621.

[14] Glehen, O., Gilly, F. N., Arvieux, C. et al. Peritoneal carcinomatosis from gastric cancer: A multi-institutional study of 159 patients treated by cytoreductive surgery combined with perioperative intraperitoneal chemotherapy. *Ann. Surg. Oncol.,* 2010; 17:2370 - 7.

[15] Gill, R. S., Al-Adra, D. P., Nagendran, J., Campbell, S., Shi, X., Haase, E., Schiller, D. Treatment of gastric cancer with peritoneal carcinomatosis by cytoreductive surgery and HIPEC: A systematic review of survival, mortality, and morbidity. *J. Surg. Oncol.,* 2011 Nov. 1; 104(6):692 - 8.

[16] Cortés-Guiral, D., Mohamed, F., Glehen, O., Passot, G. Prehabilitation of patients undergoing cytoreductive surgery (CRS) and hyperthermic intraperitoneal chemotherapy (HIPEC) for peritoneal malignancy. *Eur. J. Surg. Oncol.,* 2021 Jan.; 47(1):60 - 64.

[17] Ashvin, R., Nikhilesh, J. Preoperative Preparation and Patient Selection for Cytoreductive Surgery and HIPEC. *Indian J. Surg. Oncol.,* 2016 Jun.; 7(2):208 - 14.

[18] Hübner, M., Kusamura, S., Villeneuve, L., Al-Niaimi, A., Alyami, M., Balonov, K., Bell, J., Bristow, R., Guiral, D. C., Fagotti, A., Falcão, L. F. R., Glehen, O., Lambert, L., Mack, L., Muenster, T., Piso, P., Pocard, M., Rau, B., Sgarbura, O., Somashekhar, S. P., Wadhwa, A., Altman, A., Fawcett, W., Veerapong, J., Nelson, G.

Guidelines for Perioperative Care in Cytoreductive Surgery (CRS) with or without hyperthermic IntraPEritoneal chemotherapy (HIPEC): Enhanced recovery after surgery (ERAS®) Society Recommendations - Part I: Preoperative and intraoperative management. *Eur. J. Surg. Oncol.,* 2020 Dec.; 46(12):2292 - 2310.

[19] Musallam, K. M., Tamim, H. M., Richards, T. et al. Preoperative anaemia and postoperative outcomes in non-cardiac surgery: A retrospective cohort study. *Lancet,* 2011; 378(9800):1396e407.

[20] Kushi, L. H., Doyle, C., McCullough, M. et al. American Cancer Society guidelines on nutrition and physical activity for cancer prevention: reducing the risk of cancer withhealthy food choices and physical activity. *CA Cancer J. Clin.,* 2012; 62(1):30 - 67.

[21] Dahabreh, I. J., Steele, D. W., Shah, N., Trikalinos, T. A. Oral mechanical bowel preparation for colorectal surgery: Systematic review and meta-analysis. *Dis. Colon. Rectum*, 2015; 58(7):698e707.

[22] Koskenvuo, L., Lehtonen, T., Koskensalo, S. et al. Mechanical and oral antibiotic bowel preparation versus no bowel preparation for elective colectomy (MOBILE): A multicentre, randomised, parallel, single-blinded trial. *Lancet,* 2019; 394(10201):840e8.

[23] Practice guidelines for preoperative fasting and the use of pharmacologic agents to reduce the risk of pulmonary aspiration: Application to healthy patients undergoing elective procedures: An updated report by the American society of anesthesiologists' task force on preoperative fasting and the use of pharmacologic agents to reduce the risk of pulmonary aspiration. *Anesthesiology,* 2017; 126(3):376e93.

[24] Lu, P. W., Fields, A. C., Shabat, G., Bleday, R., Goldberg, J. E., Irani. J., Stopfkuchen-Evans, M., Melnitchouk, N. Cytoreductive Surgery and HIPEC in an Enhanced Recovery after Surgery Program: A Feasibility Study. *J. Surg. Res.,* 2020 Mar.; 247:59 - 65.

[25] Hotopp, T. HIPEC and CRS in peritoneal metastatic gastric cancer - who really benefits? *Surg. Oncol.,* 2019 Mar.; 28:159 - 166.

[26] Rudloff, U., Langan, R. C., Mullinax, J. E., Beane, J. D., Steinberg, S. M., Beresnev, T. Impact of maximal cytoreductive surgery plus

regional heated intraperitonealchemotherapy (HIPEC) on outcome of patients with peritoneal carcinomatosis of gastric origin: Results of the GYMSSA trial. *J. Surg. Oncol.,* 110 (3) (2014) 275 - 284.

[27] Glehen, O., Gilly, F. N., Arvieux, C., Cotte, E., Boutitie, F., Mansvelt, B. Peritoneal carcinomatosis from gastric cancer: a multi-institutional study of 159 patients treated by cytoreductive surgery combined with perioperative intraperitonealchemotherapy. *Ann. Surg. Oncol.,* 17 (9) (2010) 2370 - 2377.

[28] Nelson, R. L., Gladman, E., Barbateskovic, M. Antimicrobial prophylaxis for colorectal surgery. *Cochrane Database Syst. Rev.,* 2014; 5:CD001181.

In: Gastric Peritoneal Carcinomatosis ISBN: 978-1-53619-487-6
Editors: F. López Mozos et al.

Chapter 6

GASTRIC CANCER, THE MULTIDISCIPLINARY APPROACH

Marisol Huerta, MD, Valentina Gambardella, PhD and Tania Fleitas*, PhD
Hospital Clínico Universitario - Valencia, Valencia, Spain

ABSTRACT

Gastric cancer (GC) is the fifth-most common cancer worldwide and the third most common cause of cancer related-deaths worldwide. Surgery still represents the only curative approach for localized GC, but only few patients present operable disease at time of diagnosis. Moreover, even in case of curative resection, the prognosis remains poor due to the high rate of disease relapse. The current approach for localized GC patients should include the clinical assessment and staging completed by the discussion of each case into a multidisciplinary board to consider the best therapeutic. The pathological assessment and estimation of risk is mandatory for each case. The quality of surgery is essential. In this chapter we will review the most important data that support the different strategies from the classical approach to the present one.

* Corresponding Author's E-mail: tfleitask@gmail.com.

INTRODUCTION

Gastric cancer (GC) is the fifth-most common cancer worldwide and the third cause of cancer-related-death worldwide [1]. Currently, surgery still represents the only curative approach for localized GC, however, only few patients show operable disease. Sadly, even in case of curative resection, the prognosis remains poor due to the high rate of relapse [2]. For this reason, the role of a multidisciplinary board is fundamental for the staging TNM evaluation [3], the correct management and the evaluation of post-operative chemotherapy (CT) or chemo-radiation (CRT). Careful tumour staging is essential to ensure that patients are appropriately selected for treatment interventions. The recommended clinical staging tests should include at least a full blood count, liver and kidney functions, TC scan/PET scan if available, endoscopy + biopsies, endoscopic ultrasound (EUS) and staging laparoscopy. Laparoscopy ± peritoneal washings for malignant cells is recommended in all stage IB-III gastric cancers which are considered potentially resectable, to exclude radiologically occult metastatic disease; the benefit may be greater for patients with T3/T4 disease [III, B] [2].

Several meta-analyses had analysed the benefit of adjuvant CT versus surgery alone, and only limited benefit has been observed [4-8]. Moreover, it has been noted that the amount of the increase in disease-free survival was higher when adjuvant CT was administered in Asian trials [6, 8]. One of the possible causes that could justify the worsening results in western trials includes the absence of standardized surgery and the use of a less intense CT. In general, the accrual was slow, and the enrolled population was quite selected as most of them had a low risk of relapse. In the real world, many patients present a significant weight loss after total gastrectomy making them ineligible for adjuvant CT. However, a large meta-analysis of individual data of several adjuvant CT trials in GC confirmed a significant 6% absolute benefit in overall survival (OS) for 5-FU-based CT, compared with surgery alone [hazard ratio (HR) 0.82, 95% confidence interval (CI) 0.76-0.90; $P < 0.001$] in all subgroups tested [I, A] [7].

In a Korean trial, about 1000 patients diagnosed with stage II or III GC, were enrolled to receive adjuvant capecitabine plus oxaliplatin versus observation after D2 gastrectomy was conducted [9]. The planned interim analysis with a median follow-up of 34 months showed that adjuvant capecitabine plus oxaliplatin significantly improved disease-free survival (DFS), 68% versus 53%. In addition, a significant improvement in the OS was seen with a 34% decrease on the risk of death in patients treated with adjuvant CT.

Due to the high rate of local relapse after surgery, the role of post-operative radiotherapy was also studied by the American group and published by John Mc Donald in NEJM in 2001. Patients were stratified according to TNM to receive no treatment with 5Fluorouracil (5FU) alone vs 5FU and RT [10]. Despite this trial was limited by the RT technology performed and the high percentage of patients who underwent a D0-D1 dissection, the results showed an improvement for both OS and PFS for the multimodal approach. The benefit of the combination of CTRT was confirmed in the long-term analysis [11]. The improvement in relapse free and OS was confirmed with a significant decrease in loco-regional relapses coming down from 47% in the surgery only arm to 24% for the post-operative CRT arm. However, the role of post-operative radiation was not been confirmed by other studies.In the Korean phase III ARTIST trial, 458 patients were randomized between adjuvant CT with six cycles of cisplatin and capecitabine (XP) versus two cycles of XP followed by postoperative CRT including 45 Gy with concurrent capecitabine followed by two more cycles of XP [12]. Survival was not different between the 2 arms indicating so far, no value on the addition of post-operative radiation in these patients operated with D2 dissection was observed. The 3-year DFS rate showed not significant differences between the 2 arms. An exploratory analysis showed that patients with nodal involvement could have a marginal benefit from CRT.

In addition, the CRITICS trial was designed in Europe as the first trial to directly compare postoperative chemo-radiotherapy vs. peri-operative CT in patients with resectable gastric adenocarcinoma [13]. Patients were stratified according to center, histology, and tumor location. Moreover, they were randomized to receive 3 courses of pre-operative CT followed by surgery, and 3 more courses of post-operative CT in the control arm while in the experimental arm concomitant CRT was provided. The primary endpoint was the OS, and the secondary endpoints include the DFS, toxicity, and quality of life.This trial failed in the primary endpoint to show superiority of postoperative chemo-radiotherapy over postoperative CT probably related with some methodological aspects such as the number of patients who were able to receive post-operative CT: about 40% of patients in both groups did not start postoperative treatment. Moreover, some variables such as type of lymph node dissection were not balanced between both groups. So far, currently post-operative CRT after preoperative CT should be considered an experimental strategy and not standard procedure for the treatment of localized GC.

THE PERI-OPERATIVE APPROACH

The role of peri-operative CT was also investigated. In the British MAGIC trial, patients with adenocarcinoma of the lower third of the oesophagus, gastric or GEA junction tumors, with operable disease were allocated straight to surgery (in the control arm), or to receive 3 cycles of pre-operative CT based on epirubicin, cisplatin and continues infusion of 5- fluorouracil (5-FU), followed by surgery and to rather complete 3 more cycles of the same scheme of CT after surgery [14]. The primary aim of this study was OS and secondary endpoints include PFS, surgical resection and quality of life. As compared with the surgery group, the perioperative-chemotherapy group had a higher likelihood of overall survival (hazard ratio for death, 0.75; 95 percent confidence interval, 0.60 to 0.93; $P = 0.009$; five-year survival rate, 36 percent vs. 23 percent) and of progression-free survival (hazard ratio for progression, 0.66; 95 percent confidence interval, 0.53 to 0.81; $P < 0.001$). The results showed that pre-operative CT did not increase surgical related mortality nor the post-operative complications. Post-operative deaths rates were 6% for both arms and post-operative complications were observed in 46% in both groups.

There were no differences in the median duration of post-operative hospitalization neither with 13 days for both arms. Peri-operative CT was not only able to downstaging the tumor but also to translating in a significant benefit in PFS and OS becoming the standard of care in Europe. In addition, a retrospective analysis of the MAGIC trial provides relevant information on the effect on downstaging and the tumor regression grade after pre-operative CT on the surgical specimen. In fact, this analysis had shown that the presence of lymph node was the only independent predictor of survival after CT plus resection [15].

Another trial with very similar design was carried out by the French group [16]. This phase III randomized trial enrolled 224 patients with resectable tumors including the lower esophagus, the GEA junction, or stomach. Patients were randomly assigned to either peri-operative cisplatin/5FU and surgery thereafter or surgery alone. The experimental arm had a better OS with a decrease in the risk of death of 31% as well as a better DFS (5-year rate: 34% v 19%; HR, 0.65).

The Current Peri-Operative Approach

According to international guidelines [2, 17], all patients with stage IB to III gastric adenocarcinoma would benefit form a systemic. For those patients going straight to surgery if a D2 dissection was done adjuvant CT could be an option. In patients in whom a D2 dissection was not performed, post-operative CT or concurrent CRT is indicated. However, peri-operative CT is the preferred approach in Europe due to the outcomes seeing in the MAGIC and the FLOT-4 trials.

The European standard of care is currently based on the FLOT-4 trial [18], a phase II/III academic randomized German study. More than 700 patients with GC and GEJ adenocarcinoma were included. They were stratified according to the ECOG, tumor location, age, and nodal status. Patients were randomized to receive peri-operative CT with 2 different arms: the control arm was the standard of care based on the MAGIC trial (3 cycles of ECF or ECX followed by surgery and other 3 more cycles);

and the experimental arm, a new scheme including docetaxel, oxaliplatin, continuous infusion of 5 FU during 24 hours and leucovorin. The results showed a median OS of 35 months for the control arm, versus 50 months achieved with FLOT (HR = 0.77). The toxicity, it was similar for both arms, and the detected toxicities were moderate, mostly grades 1-2. For the control arm nausea, vomiting, anaemia and thromboembolic events were the most common; while in the FLOT arm, the most frequent adverse events were diarrhoea, neutropenia, infections and the neurotoxicity related with oxaliplatin. FLOT-4 regimen not only showed a great benefit in OS but also in inducing pathological response, showing 15,6% pathological response rates. Remarkably, this trial was a gamechanger and the level of evidence of the results was A, according to the magnitude of benefit of the ESMO magnitude scale, due to the 9% increase in the median OS for 5 years.

THE ROLE OF PRE-OPERATIVE CHEMORADIATION

The role of pre-operative CRT is under evaluation in an open label randomized controlled multi-center international study: the TOP GEAR study [18]. In this, patients with locally advanced esophageal, gastric, or gastro esophageal (GEA) adenocarcinoma are randomized to perioperative CT (ECF or similar schedules or even FLOT) as the control arm or to an experimental arm in which CRT is added. The primary endpoint is DFS, and the secondary endpoints include the OS, the pattern and rate of relapse, the loco-regional and distant failure, safety and quality of life.

For GEA junction tumours, the role of pre-operative CRT derives from the Dutch CROSS trial [19]. In this study, 275 patients were recruited, diagnosed with oesophageal and GEA junction adenocarcinoma (in addition to 84 squamous cell carcinoma patients), the combination of radiotherapy with 5 weeks of weekly paclitaxel and carboplatin versus surgery alone was compared. Patients treated with the experimental arm showed a significant improvement in R0 resection rates (92% versus 69%) and OS (3-year overall survival 58% vs. 44%). A recent update to the long-term survival results of the CROSS trial suggests that the incidence of distant metastases is also reduced by CRT for up to 2 years following surgery [HR 0.63, p = 0.0040] [20]· Based on the results of the FLOT-4and the CROSS study, we can conclude that for Western countries, both options could be considered as peri-operative strategy in GEJ adenocarcinomas [2].

The locoregional approach consisting in intraperitoneal CT or HIPEC have also been validated in several trials [21-23]. Nevertheless, the results of those are not conclusive across Western population [2]. A large French series demonstrated a median survival of surgery plus HIPEC of 9.2 months, with a 5-year survival rate of 13% for all patients and 23% for those who had complete cytoreductive surgery [24]. Further validation is awaited.

Immunotherapy for Gastric Cancer

The comprehensive molecular and functional characterization of the Cancer Genome Atlas (TCGA) classification has established four main gastric cancer subgroups: Epstein Barr virus (EBV) positive cancers, tumors with microsatellite instability (MSI), genomic stability (GS) and chromosomal instability (CIN) [25]. However, this classification has no prognostic value. Nevertheless, patients with MSI do have a better prognosis across stages I-III compared with the other subgroups, so that the role of CT is not clear. In a study performed in our institution [26], the 10 Y median OS for the MSI group was 80% while it was 50% for the MSS group. To address if perioperative CT could benefit patients with MSI-GC, a retrospective analysis from the MAGIC trial was performed. Patients with MSI profile benefit from surgery alone. However, a negative effect was observed for MSI-patients treated with peri-operative CT followed by surgery, indicating that patients with MSI would not benefit from this strategy [27]. In another study carried out by Korean investigators in the CLASSIC study, similar observations were found, patients with MSI treated with post-operative CT based on capecitabine and oxaliplatin, didn´t showed any improvement comparing the group treated with surgery alone with a median 5 years OS of about 80% for both groups. However, patients with MSS do benefit from the addition of post-operative CT [28]. These data suggest that MSS status should be analyzed to consider which patients could benefit from the addition of CT for localized GC.

The phase III trial Checkmate 577 trial [29] has showed interesting results. This study randomized patients diagnosed with stage II/III esophageal and GEJ adenocarcinoma, who were previously treated with neoadjuvant chemoradiation + surgery, to receive adjuvant nivolumab vs placebo up to 1 year. Nivolumab provided superior DFS with a 31% reduction in the risk of recurrence or death (p = 00003) and a doubling in median DFS versus placebo, with an acceptable toxicity profile, and without detrimental in the quality of life.

The VESTIGE study [30] (NCT03443856), is an open randomized multicenter phase II study planned for patients with poor regression after neoadjuvant CT. Patients with positive lymph nodes and/or tumor involved resection margin, can be included in this study. They are randomized to receive immunotherapy (combining Nivolumab, a PD-1 immune check-point inhibitor, associated with the CTLA4 inhibitor Ipilimumab) vs CT according to the standard of care. The primary endpoint is DFS. The recruitment of this trial is ongoing at this moment.

Finally, the research is focusing on the role of immunotherapy for GC in the perioperative setting. Currently ongoing, the Phase III KEYNOTE-585 study (NCT03221426) seeks to evaluate the efficacy and safety of pembrolizumab plus chemotherapy, compared with placebo plus chemotherapy (according to CF or FLOT-4 schedule), as a perioperative treatment for localized gastric or GEJ adenocarcinoma. The Phase I/II ICONIC trial (NCT03399071), evaluate the safety and efficacy of avelumab in combination with FLOT-4 [31].

OTHER EXPERIMENTAL APPROACHES

A randomized international trial (TOGA trial) enrolling HER2 amplified patients diagnosed with locally advanced or metastatic GC was conducted to evaluate trastuzumab plus chemotherapy (capecitabine, cisplatin) versus chemotherapy alone in HER2+ advanced gastric and GEA patients. Significant improvement in overall survival (OS) (13.8 vs. 11.1 months, Hazard ratio [HR] 0.74, p = 0.0046), progression-free survival (PFS) (6.7 vs. 5.5 months, HR 0.71, p = 0.0002), and overall response rate (ORR) (47% vs. 35%, p = 0.0017) was underlined among patients treated with the experimental arm. For this reason, since 2010, the combination of trastuzumab + platinum-based chemotherapy represents the golden standard for *HER2* amplified patients for the frontline of the metastatic setting [32].

For HER2 positive localized GC patients, the benefit of the addition of anti-Her2 therapy is currently under evaluation. The PETRARCA study [33] was a phase 2/3 study including patients with GEA adenocarcinomas T2-4 N0/N+, HER2 positive, who were randomized to receive standard FLOT vs perioperative FLOT + trastuzumab and pertuzumab and trastuzumab and pertuzumab as maintenance treatment x 9 cycles. This study was ended early, because of the results of the JACOB study in the metastatic setting [34], but the results from 81 patients included in the phase 2 part of the PETRARCA trial showed promising results: a significant improvement in the pathological response rates (primary endpoint) from 12% (FLOT arm) to 35% in the combination arm p = 0.02. Another academic study that is evaluating the HER2 strategy is the INNOVATION study, guided by the EORTC group [35] (NCT02205047). This trial is currently under recruitment and randomize patients to three different arms FLOT vs FLOT + trastuzumab vs FLOT + trastuzumab and pertuzumab.

The combination of antiangiogenics and CT was also tested in the peri-operative setting. Bevacizumab (anti VEGF1) added to capecitabine + cisplatin + epirubicin regimen [36] failed to demonstrate a benefit in the OS in a phase II/III randomized trial including more than 1000 patients. In addition, bevacizumab was also associated with impaired wound healing in this study. Ramucirumab (anti-VEGFR2 antibody) was also tested added to FLOT-4 chemotherapy in the perioperative setting vs FLOT in the RAMSES- FLOT-7 phase II study [37], including 180 patients. The primary endpoint was focused on the complete pathological rate and R0 resection. No difference in path response rates was seen between FLOT, 30% and FLOT-RAM, 27%. However, FLOT-RAM significantly improved R0-resection rate (FLOT, 82%; FLOT-RAM, 96%, p = 0.0078). Patients with Siewert type I adenocarcinoma were excluded from the study because of safety reasons. Benefit of FLOT-RAM was more meaningful for the cT3/T4 group (FLOT, 80%; FLOT-RAM, 97%), and the diffuse/mixed histology (FLOT, 77%; FLOT-RAM, 95%).

Considerations for the Elderly Population

The definition of an "elderly patient" varies according to the different geographic areas. Aging is associated with an increase in comorbidity, as well as an increased incidence of cancer. All these, could cause a change in pharmacodynamic and pharmacokinetics, with an increased toxicity. A comprehensive geriatric assessment (CGA) is a useful method to assess life expectancy and risk of morbidity and mortality in older patients. Based on the result of the CGA, physicians can estimate the risk and benefits of anti-cancer treatment in the individual patient, especially considering "surgery" as the main aim of the therapeutic approach for resectable GC and EGJ adenocarcinoma. Hurria et al., [38] developed a brief CGA specific for elderly patients with cancer, Cancer-Specific Geriatric Assessment (CSGA). It assesses elderly patients using seven domains including functional status, comorbidity, polypharmacy, cognitive function, psychological status, social functioning and support, and nutritional status. Moreover, it´s also important to consider that in most of the clinical trials limited information could be found for the elderly population, and for this reason perioperative chemotherapy needs to be considered on an individual basis for elderly patients 70 years or older [39].

CONCLUSION

GC is a complex disease; thus, a multidisciplinary team approach is necessary to offer an optimal management. Perioperative CT do induce downstaging, may increase the R0 resection rate, prolongs disease free survival improves OS and provided evidence level I based upon 2 well designed and properly conducted randomised trials adjuvant treatment is cc However, preoperative therapy is better tolerated than postoperatively. The quality of surgery is essential and the management of localized GC. Postoperative CRT has limited value if D2 surgery was performed or preoperative CT was given. Preoperative CRT is under scrutiny in TOPGEAR trial. MSI high tumour do not seem to do benefit the most from adjuvant or neoadjuvant CT. Despite the promising results, the use of checkpoint inhibitor as adjuvant treatment still not represents the standard of care. The addition of HER2 inhibitors in this setting is still under investigation. Further research on biological predictive factors is needed.

REFERENCES

[1] Bray F., Ferlay J., Soerjomataram I. et al., Global cancer statistics 2018: GLOBOCAN estimates of incidence and mortality worldwide for 36 cancers in 185 countries. *CA Cancer J Clin* 2018; 68: 394-424.

[2] Smyth E. C., Verheij M., Allum W. et al., Gastric cancer: ESMO Clinical Practice Guidelines for diagnosis, treatment and follow-up. *Ann Oncol* 2016; 27: v38-v49.

[3] O'Sullivan B., Brierley J., Byrd D. et al., The TNM classification of malignant tumours-towards common understanding and reasonable expectations. *Lancet Oncol* 2017; 18: 849-851.

[4] Earle C. C., Maroun J. A. Adjuvant chemotherapy after curative resection for gastric cancer in non-Asian patients: revisiting a meta-analysis of randomised trials. *European Journal of Cancer* 1999; 35: 1059-1064.

[5] Janunger K. G., Hafström L., Glimelius B. Chemotherapy in gastric cancer: a review and updated meta-analysis. *Eur J Surg* 2002; 168: 597-608.

[6] Zhao S. L., Fang J. Y. The role of postoperative adjuvant chemotherapy following curative resection for gastric cancer: a meta-analysis. *Cancer Invest* 2008; 26: 317-325.

[7] Paoletti X., Oba K., Burzykowski T. et al., Benefit of adjuvant chemotherapy for resectable gastric cancer: a meta-analysis. *Jama* 2010; 303: 1729-1737.

[8] Liu T. S., Wang Y., Chen S. Y., Sun Y. H. An updated meta-analysis of adjuvant chemotherapy after curative resection for gastric cancer. *Eur J Surg Oncol* 2008; 34: 1208-1216.

[9] Noh S. H., Park S. R., Yang H. K. et al., Adjuvant capecitabine plus oxaliplatin for gastric cancer after D2 gastrectomy (CLASSIC): 5-year follow-up of an open-label, randomised phase 3 trial. *Lancet Oncol* 2014; 15: 1389-1396.

[10] Macdonald J. S., Smalley S. R., Benedetti J. et al., Chemoradiotherapy after surgery compared with surgery alone for adenocarcinoma of the stomach or gastroesophageal junction. *N Engl J Med* 2001; 345: 725-730.

[11] Smalley S. R., Benedetti J. K., Haller D. G. et al., Updated Analysis of SWOG-Directed Intergroup Study 0116: A Phase III Trial of Adjuvant Radiochemotherapy Versus Observation After Curative Gastric Cancer Resection. *Journal of Clinical Oncology* 2012; 30: 2327-2333.

[12] Park S. H., Sohn T. S., Lee J. et al., Phase III Trial to Compare Adjuvant Chemotherapy with Capecitabine and Cisplatin Versus Concurrent Chemoradiotherapy in Gastric Cancer: Final Report of the Adjuvant Chemoradiotherapy in Stomach Tumors Trial, Including Survival and Subset Analyses. *Journal of clinical oncology: official journal of the American Society of Clinical Oncology* 2015; 33: 3130-3136.

[13] Cats A., Jansen E. P. M., van Grieken N. C. T. et al., Chemotherapy versus chemoradiotherapy after surgery and preoperative

chemotherapy for resectable gastric cancer (CRITICS): an international, open-label, randomised phase 3 trial. *Lancet Oncol* 2018; 19: 616-628.

[14] Cunningham D., Allum W. H., Stenning S. P. et al., Perioperative chemotherapy versus surgery alone for resectable gastroesophageal cancer. *N Engl J Med* 2006; 355: 11-20.

[15] Smyth E. C., Fassan M., Cunningham D. et al., Effect of Pathologic Tumor Response and Nodal Status on Survival in the Medical Research Council Adjuvant Gastric Infusional Chemotherapy Trial. *J Clin Oncol* 2016; 34: 2721-2727.

[16] Ychou M., Boige V., Pignon J. P. et al., Perioperative chemotherapy compared with surgery alone for resectable gastroesophageal adenocarcinoma: an FNCLCC and FFCD multicenter phase III trial. *J Clin Oncol* 2011; 29: 1715-1721.

[17] Wagner A. D., Lordick F., Grabsch H. I. et al., Multidisciplinary management of stage II-III gastric and gastro-oesophageal junction cancer. *Eur J Cancer* 2020; 124: 67-76.

[18] Al-Batran S. E., Homann N., Pauligk C. et al., Perioperative chemotherapy with fluorouracil plus leucovorin, oxaliplatin, and docetaxel versus fluorouracil or capecitabine plus cisplatin and epirubicin for locally advanced, resectable gastric or gastro-oesophageal junction adenocarcinoma (FLOT4): a randomised, phase 2/3 trial. *Lancet* 2019; 393: 1948-1957.

[19] van Hagen P., Hulshof M. C., van Lanschot J. J. et al., Preoperative chemoradiotherapy for esophageal or junctional cancer. *N Engl J Med* 2012; 366: 2074-2084.

[20] Shapiro J., van Lanschot J. J. B., Hulshof M. et al., Neoadjuvant chemoradiotherapy plus surgery versus surgery alone for oesophageal or junctional cancer (CROSS): long-term results of a randomised controlled trial. *Lancet Oncol* 2015; 16: 1090-1098.

[21] Fujimoto S., Takahashi M., Mutou T. et al., Successful intraperitoneal hyperthermic chemoperfusion for the prevention of postoperative peritoneal recurrence in patients with advanced gastric carcinoma. *Cancer* 1999; 85: 529-534.

[22] Fujimura T., Yonemura Y., Muraoka K. et al., Continuous hyperthermic peritoneal perfusion for the prevention of peritoneal recurrence of gastric cancer: randomized controlled study. *World J Surg* 1994; 18: 150-155.
[23] Yang X. J., Huang C. Q., Suo T. et al., Cytoreductive surgery and hyperthermic intraperitoneal chemotherapy improves survival of patients with peritoneal carcinomatosis from gastric cancer: final results of a phase III randomized clinical trial. *Ann Surg Oncol* 2011; 18: 1575-1581.
[24] Glehen O., Gilly F. N., Arvieux C. et al., Peritoneal carcinomatosis from gastric cancer: a multi-institutional study of 159 patients treated by cytoreductive surgery combined with perioperative intraperitoneal chemotherapy. *Ann Surg Oncol* 2010; 17: 2370-2377.
[25] Cancer Genome Atlas Research N. Comprehensive molecular characterization of gastric adenocarcinoma. *Nature* 2014; 513: 202-209.
[26] Martinez-Ciarpaglini C., Fleitas-Kanonnikoff T., Gambardella V. et al., Assessing molecular subtypes of gastric cancer: microsatellite unstable and Epstein-Barr virus subtypes. Methods for detection and clinical and pathological implications. *ESMO Open* 2019; 4: e000470.
[27] Smyth E. C., Wotherspoon A., Peckitt C. et al., Mismatch Repair Deficiency, Microsatellite Instability, and Survival: An Exploratory Analysis of the Medical Research Council Adjuvant Gastric Infusional Chemotherapy (MAGIC) Trial. *JAMA Oncol* 2017; 3: 1197-1203.
[28] Choi Y. Y., Kim H., Shin S. J. et al., Microsatellite Instability and Programmed Cell Death-Ligand 1 Expression in Stage II/III Gastric Cancer: Post Hoc Analysis of the CLASSIC Randomized Controlled study. *Ann Surg* 2019; 270: 309-316.
[29] Jaa R. J. K., J. Kuzdzal, T. Zander, E. Van Cutsem, G. Piessen, G. Mendez, J. L. Feliciano, S. Motoyama, A. Lièvre, H. Uronis, E. Elimova, C. Grootscholten, K. Geboes, J. Zhang, L. Zhu, M. Lei, K. Kondo, J. M. Cleary, M. Moehler. Adjuvant nivolumab in resected

esophageal or gastroesophageal junction cancer (EC/GEJC) following neoadjuvant chemoradiation therapy (CRT): First results of the CheckMate 577 study. *In Annals of Oncology* (2020) 31 (suppl_4): S1142-S1215. https://10.1016/annonc/annonc325. 2020.

[30] Smyth E., Knödler M., Giraut A. et al., VESTIGE: Adjuvant Immunotherapy in Patients With Resected Esophageal, Gastroesophageal Junction and Gastric Cancer Following Preoperative Chemotherapy With High Risk for Recurrence (N+ and/or R1): An Open Label Randomized Controlled Phase-2-Study. *Front Oncol* 2019; 9: 1320.

[31] Petrillo A., Pompella L., Tirino G. et al., Perioperative Treatment in Resectable Gastric Cancer: Current Perspectives and Future Directions. *Cancers* (Basel) 2019; 11.

[32] Bang Y. J., Van Cutsem E., Feyereislova A. et al., Trastuzumab in combination with chemotherapy versus chemotherapy alone for treatment of HER2-positive advanced gastric or gastro-oesophageal junction cancer (ToGA): a phase 3, open-label, randomised controlled trial. *Lancet* 2010; 376: 687-697.

[33] Al-Batran S., G. M. Haag, T. J. Ettrich, K. Borchert, A. Kretzschmar, C. Teschendorf, G. M. Siegler, M. Ebert, E. Goekkurt, M. K. Welslau, R. J. C. Mahlberg, N. Homann, D. Pink, W. O. Bechstein, P. Reichardt T. Gaiser, D. Sookthai, C. Pauligk, T. O. Goetze, R. D. Hofheinz. Final results and subgroup analysis of the PETRARCA randomized phase II AIO trial: Perioperative trastuzumab and pertuzumab in combination with FLOT versus FLOT alone for HER2 positive resectable esophagogastric adenocarcinoma. *In Annals of Oncology* (2020) 31 (suppl_4): S841-S873. https://10.1016/annonc/annonc284.2020.

[34] Tabernero J., Hoff P. M., Shen L. et al., Pertuzumab plus trastuzumab and chemotherapy for HER2-positive metastatic gastric or gastro-oesophageal junction cancer (JACOB): final analysis of a double-blind, randomised, placebo-controlled phase 3 study. *Lancet Oncol* 2018; 19: 1372-1384.

[35] Wagner A. D., Grabsch H. I., Mauer M. et al., EORTC-1203-GITCG - the "Innovation"-trial: Effect of chemotherapy alone versus chemotherapy plus trastuzumab, versus chemotherapy plus trastuzumab plus pertuzumab, in the perioperative treatment of HER2 positive, gastric and gastroesophageal junction adenocarcinoma on pathologic response rate: a randomized phase II-intergroup trial of the EORTC-Gastrointestinal Tract Cancer Group, Korean Cancer Study Group and Dutch Upper GI-Cancer group. *BMC Cancer* 2019; 19: 494.

[36] Comprehensive molecular characterization of gastric adenocarcinoma. *Nature* 2014; 513: 202-209.

[37] Al-Batran S., R. D. Hofheinz, H. Schmalenberg, D. Strumberg, E. Goekkurt, S. Angermeier, T. Zander, J. Potenberg, H. Kopp, D. Pink, G. M. Siegler, M. Schenk, F. De Vita, E. Maiello, T. Gaiser, D. Sookthai, U. S. Bankstahl, C. Pauligk, T. O. Götze, N. Homann. Perioperative FLOT plus ramucirumab versus FLOT alone for resectable esophagogastric adenocarcinoma – Updated results and subgroup analyses of the randomized phase II/III trial RAMSES/FLOT7 of the German AIO and Italian GOIM. In *Annals of Oncology* (2020) 31 (suppl_4): S841-S873. https://10.1016/annonc/annonc284. 2020.

[38] Hurria A., Gupta S., Zauderer M. et al., Developing a cancer-specific geriatric assessment: a feasibility study. *Cancer* 2005; 104: 1998-2005.

[39] Kim H. S., Kim J. H., Kim J. W., Kim B. C. Chemotherapy in Elderly Patients with Gastric Cancer. *J Cancer* 2016; 7: 88-94.

In: Gastric Peritoneal Carcinomatosis
Editors: F. López Mozos et al.
ISBN: 978-1-53619-487-6

Chapter 7

PATHOPHYSIOLOGIC BASIS, PRINCIPLES AND TECHNIQUE OF CYTOREDUCTIVE SURGERY (CRS) FOR GASTRIC CANCER PERITONEAL METASTASES

P. Barrios*, MD, PhD, I. Ramos, MD and L. Bijelic, MD
Compleix Hospitalari Moisès Broggi
Sant Joan Despí, Barcelona, Spain

ABSTRACT

In this chapter we will discuss the role of radical combined treatment of peritoneal carcinomatosis (CRS+HIPEC). Specific features of peritoneal metastases from gastric cancer, the importance of the tumor biology, the impact on the selection of patients according to the PCI score and possibilities of performing a CC-0 resection are discussed. We will highlight the abdomino-pelvic areas with the greatest possibilities of being affected, the preoperative estimation of peritoneal metastases and surgical radicality, as well as the importance of the detection of non-

* Corresponding Author's E-mail: pedro.barrios@sanitatintegral.org.

accessible lesions and the role of preoperative laparoscopy for staging purpose. Peritonectomy procedures and other requested techniques are described (video demonstration in the eBook version), including comments on the minimally invasive approach. We describe the most frequent postoperative complications and finally present authors' results.

INTRODUCTION

Peritoneal seeding is one of the most common patterns of gastric cancer dissemination [1]. Autopsy studies show that 50-60% of patients who die due to gastric cancer have peritoneal progression and evidence of carcinomatosis at the time of death [2, 3]. Among patients with newly diagnosed gastric cancer, the incidence of peritoneal involvement is 14%. Overall, the peritoneum is the only site of metastases in 10% of gastric cancer patients and among those who recur after initial curative intent surgery, the peritoneum is involved in 12-40% [4].

Compared to peritoneal metastases of other gastrointestinal origins, gastric cancer carcinomatosis shows specific morphological and biological characteristics that influence both the indications and inclusion criteria for cytoreductive surgery (with heated intraperitoneal chemotherapy) as well as some technical aspects of the surgery.

THE INFLUENCE OF TUMOR BIOLOGY IN THE NATURAL HISTORY OF GASTRIC CANCER

The natural history of gastric cancer is determined by the biology and behaviour of gastric cancer malignant cells. The shedding of neoplastic cells into the free abdominal cavity is common and can occur spontaneously from the surface of an advanced primary tumor that has penetrated the visceral peritoneum, due to tumor perforation or by extravasation of malignant cells from blood vessels and lymphatics that have been opened during surgery. These free cancer cells (FCCs) can generate a cascade of events that begins with an interaction with the mesothelial layer of the peritoneum and eventually leads to a diffuse macroscopic involvement of the peritoneal lining and abdominal organs by carcinomatosis. The aggressive biologic behavior of gastric FCCs in the peritoneal fluid determines the classification of positive peritoneal cytology as M1 disease due to its prognostic significance similar to macroscopic peritoneal metastases [5, 8]. More recently, the detection of molecular markers indicative of the presence of malignant cells in the peritoneal fluid has been used as a complementary method of peritoneal fluid assessment that complements the traditional cytological examination [9].

The distribution of FCCs in the abdominal cavity is influenced by the dynamic characteristics of peritoneal fluid flow and its relationship with the anatomic and functional characteristics of the abdominal organs and structures.

Furthermore, the peritoneal surface contains microscopic structures named "lymphatic stomata" that allow the penetration of malignant cells into the mesothelial layer where molecular interactions that favor implantation and tumor progression can occur. Some regions of the peritoneal cavity are characterized by a greater concentration of lymphatic stomata and therefore are more prone to harbor peritoneal tumor deposit. These "high risk" areas need to be well known to the peritoneal malignancy surgeon and thoroughly inspected in patients at risk of harboring gastric cancer peritoneal metastases.

Clinical Manifestations of Gastric Cancer Peritoneal Metastases

The metastatic efficiency of gastric FCCs can explain some clinical manifestations of gastric cancer carcinomatosis such as the confluent diffuse covering of the small bowel serosa and mesentery that can be seen in some advanced cases not suitable to cytoreductive surgery (Figure 1).

This form of gastric cancer peritoneal involvement also shows an infiltrating reticular pattern on the diaphragmatic and pelvic peritoneum that often times infiltrates the underlying muscular layer and other anatomical structures (Figure 2 and 3).

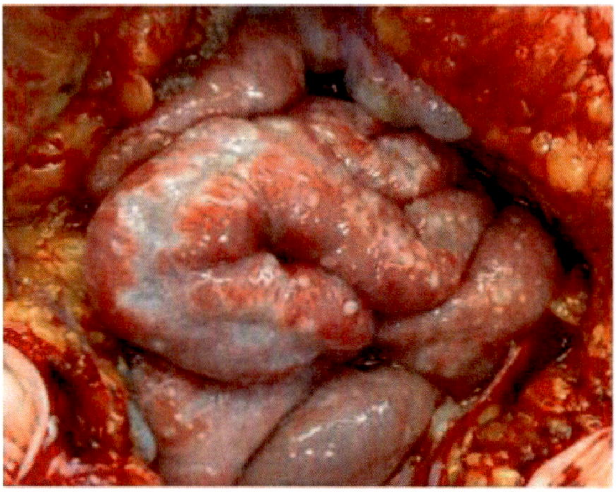

Figure 1. Diffuse involvement of small bowell serosa and the mesentery.

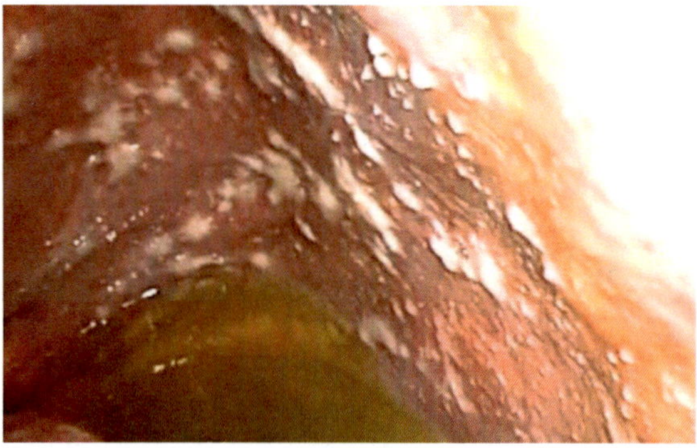

Figure 2. Right hemidiaphragm diffuse infiltrating nodules.

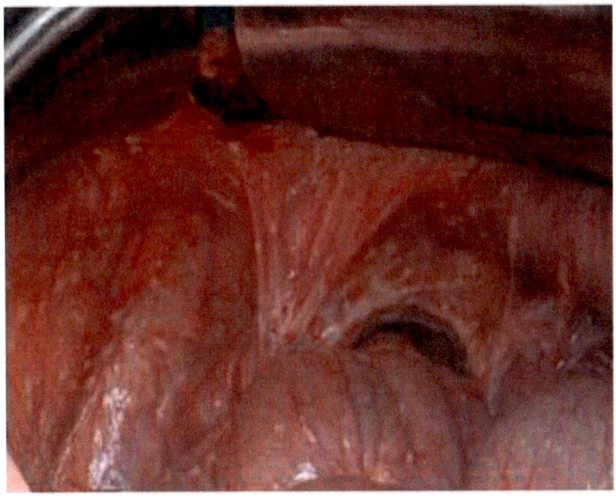

Figure 3. Infiltrating nodules involving the pelvic peritoneum.

However, the pattern most often observed in patients that may be candidates for surgical cytoreduction is characterized by the presence of multiple small to moderately sized, invasive tumor nodules with a solid, pearled appearance. They tend to be scattered through the peritoneum with a predilection for the supramesocolic compartment and the pelvic floor. The small bowel can also be involved, frequently with invasive nodules localized at the border between the bowel and its mesentery, which require special consideration due to their prognostic relevance and surgical considerations. Their tendency to progress to bowel obstruction is marked and they require of specific cytoreductive techniques (Figure 4 and 5). In the pelvis, larger or more invasive nodules can involve the wall of the rectum and those located along the pericolic sulcus can infiltrate and obstruct the ureters requiring resection and reconstruction of both structure. Cytoreduction in these instances may be indicated and feasible, as long as there are no other contraindications (Figure 6).

Occasionally, peritoneal metastases of gastric cancer can be unresectable and unsuitable for CRS and HIPEC due to their location and infiltrative nature despite a low peritoneal burden of disease. This is the case for involvement of the liver hilum, the base of the transverse colon mesentery or bilateral infiltration of pelvic sidewalls.

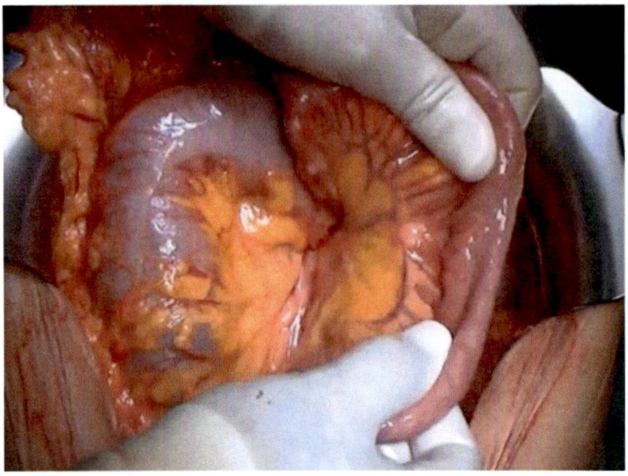

Figure 4. Mesenteric nodules without small bowel involvement.

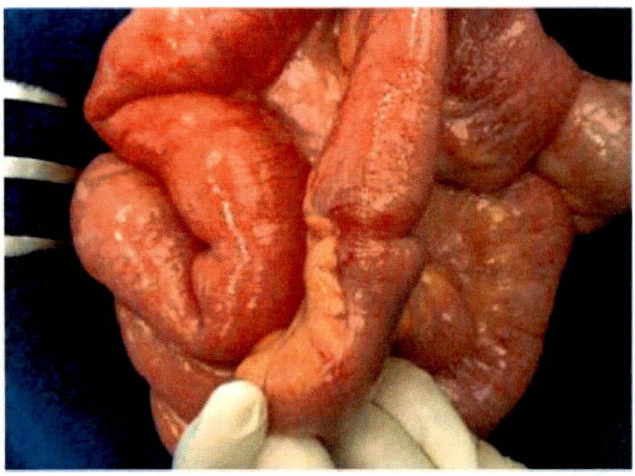

Figure 5. Nodule on the mesenteric border causing intestinal obstruction.

In addition to the extension, location and invasiveness of the peritoneal metastases, an important factor that affects the inclusion criteria for CRS and HIPEC in gastric cancer is the histology of the tumor. In patients with one or more characteristics bordering relative contraindications (such as peritoneal cancer index (PCI) near the upper acceptable limit, the need for additional visceral resections such as rectosigmoid colectomy or ureteral resection etc.) the presence of signet ring histology should be viewed as a poor prognostic sign and the indication for CRS evaluated with caution [10]. The negative prognostic influence of signet ring histology after CRS and HIPEC has been demonstrated most significantly in colon cancer where it is considered a relative contraindication to the procedure [11].

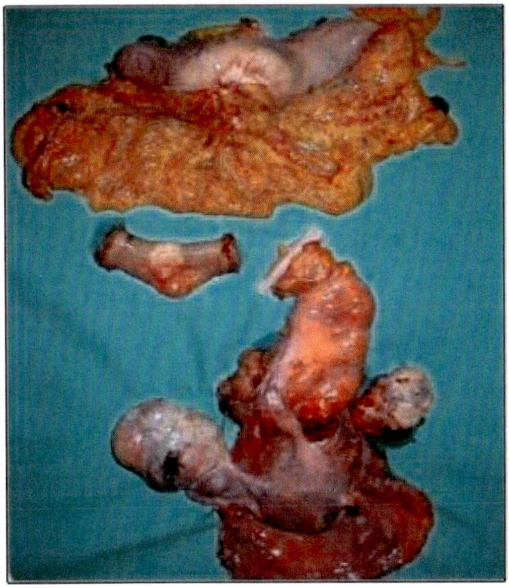

Figure 6. Resectable multivisceral peritoneal disease. PCI 11/39 (involvement of a segment of small bowell involvement, bilateral ovarian metastases-Krukenberg´s tumor, sigmoid colon and pelvic peritoneum involvement).

Preoperative Evaluation and Patient Selection for CRS and HIPEC in Gastric Cancer Peritoneal Metastases

The current indications for CRS and HIPEC in gastric cancer peritoneal metastases are based on the results of clinical studies of various levels of evidence.

The existing studies are generally similar in their inclusion criteria that emphasize the need for strict patient selection considering several factors: response to neoadjuvant chemotherapy, extent of peritoneal disease and ability to perform complete surgical resection both of the primary tumor and its associated lymphatic drainage as well as the complete macroscopic resection (CC-0) of the peritoneal disease.

Response to Neoadjuvant Systemic Chemotherapy

Evaluation of gastric cancer peritoneal metastases by imaging is limited and the application of RECIST criteria can be very difficult or impossible [12]. This is an important consideration when evaluating response to neoadjuvant chemotherapy.

The use of neoadjuvant chemotherapy prior to consideration of CRS and HIPEC in gastric cancer is considered essential. Progression during neoadjuvant chemotherapy is a contraindication to further surgical treatment. Radiological assessment of response is limited not only by the general characteristics of peritoneal metastases but also by the changes that can occur in gastric cancer peritoneal metastases during treatment. They can become more fibrotic and flat and thus even less visible by radiologic techniques. This type of response can also cause the implants to become difficult to detect during surgical exploration and to assess pathologically.

Considering the limitations of imaging techniques, laparoscopy is an important tool both for the initial diagnosis of low volume peritoneal metastases in patients with gastric cancer [13, 14] as well as for the assessment of response after neoadjuvant chemotherapy for patients who are potential candidates for CRS and HIPEC. The role of laparoscopy in these patients is twofold. The initial diagnostic and staging laparoscopy is used to diagnose the peritoneal metastases and determine their location and extent. A repeat laparoscopy after completion of neoadjuvant chemotherapy is used to determine response and rule out possible progression of disease not detectable by standard imaging.

The PCI used to include or exclude patients for CRS and HIPEC is the one seen during the initial diagnostic/staging laparosocopy.

Presence of Other Metastatic Sites

In patients with peritoneal metastases of other gastrointestinal tumors, such as colon cancer, the presence of other resectable systemic metastases (liver or pulmonary) does not represent an absolute contraindication to CRS and HIPEC. However, in gastric cancer, there is no available data that supports surgical resection in cases of metastatic disease involving multiple sites and conceptually, considering the biology of gastric cancer, the presence of systemic metastases is considered an absolute contraindication to CRS and HIPEC.

It is therefore essential to perform complete staging of patients prior to consideration of CRS.

Extent and Distribution of Peritoneal Metastases

The extent of peritoneal metastases is a key selection and prognostic factor in patients with gastric cancer. The Japanese Research Society for Gastric Cancer classified peritoneal metastases from gastric cancer according to the location and extent of the peritoneal disease [15]. Several studies have demonstrated correspondence between survival of patients with gastric carcinomatosis and peritoneal involvement with this classification system [16-18]. Other classification systems have been developed to quantify the burden of peritoneal disease [19-21] but the most validated and widely used is the PCI [22]. A modification of this quantification tool has been developed for radiological evaluation of tumor burden by CT (CT PCI). The PCI has been shown to independently predict survival in patients with peritoneal metastases of all origins including gastric cancer [23-25].

Because of its prognostic value, the radiological (and intraoperative) PCI has been used as a selection tool for CRS and HIPEC with cutoff values adjusted to the biological aggressiveness of the tumor. In tumors with an indolent biology such as mucinous appendiceal neoplasms that cause pseudomyxoma peritonei, there is no upper limit of PCI that is considered and absolute contraindication to CRS. However, in more invasive and aggressive tumors such as colon or gastric cancer, a cutoff value is often considered as a contraindication to CRS and HIPEC because patients with higher tumor burden do not show benefit after CRS and HIPEC even if a complete resection can be obtained.

Several studies have shown benefit of CRS+HIPEC in patients with peritoneal metastases of gastric cancer and a PCI of <12, <10 and <6. In practice, the most commonly utilized PCI cutoff value is a PCI <10. Patients with a higher volume of disease have poor survival rates despite complete cytoreduction and are therefore not considered candidates for the treatment [26].

Completeness of Cytoreduction Score

The ability of achieving complete macroscopic resection of disease is essential for patients undergoing surgery for gastric cancer peritoneal metastases and a strong determinant of survival.

The most commonly utilized score to quantify residual peritoneal disease following cytoreduction is the Completeness of Cytoreduction Score (CC Score). It is the strongest predictor of survival in patients undergoing cytoreductive surgery of all origins including gastric cancer [25-27].

The addition of HIPEC to CRS is closely linked to the amount of residual tumor in the abdomen following CRS. In less aggressive tumors, cytoreduction is considered complete if there is no visible residual tumor (CC-0) or if the size of residual nodules is <2.5 mm (CC-1) taking into consideration that intraperitoneal chemotherapy can penetrate into tumor deposits up to a depth of 2.5 mm. However, in more aggressive tumors such as gastric cancer, characterized by more solid and fibrotic nodules, only a CC-0 cytoreduction is considered complete since it is unlikely that intraperitoneal chemotherapy can have sufficient penetration into residual macroscopic nodules and because of significant differences in survival between patients undergoing CC-0 versus CC-1 cytoreduction.

While the probability of performing a CC-0 cytoreduction should be evaluated preoperatively as part of the selection process, the final assessment of the CC score is done intraoperatively. In some cases, the decision to proceed or not with cytoreduction in gastric cancer carcinomatosis is difficult and can only be done intraoperatively, based on a thorough exploration of the abdominal cavity and taking into consideration some peculiarities of this form of carcinomatosis. This is especially true when evaluating the small bowel and its mesentery, which can represent the limiting step in achieving a CC-0 cytoreduction. Any residual disease in this location will lead to early progression, frequently in the form of bowel obstruction and a very short symptom-free interval that does not justify the performance of any other resections during the cytoreduction.

The complete evaluation of the risks and benefits when considering proceeding with CRS and HIPEC in patients with gastric cancer peritoneal metastases has to consider the expected survival advantage of surgical resection but also the technical abilities and experience of the surgical team. In the majority of centers that perform CRS and HIPEC for peritoneal metastases, patients with gastric cancer represent a small percentage of the total cases. In fact, few single institutions have published series larger than 40 patients undergoing CRS and HIPEC for gastric carcinomatosis. The presence of advanced surgical skills and experience to treat gastric cancer peritoneal metastases are even more important than in other types of peritoneal metastases [28, 29].

In our center, of the total number of 1300 performed CRS and HIPEC cases over 14 years, gastric cancer carcinomatosis was the indication in only 58 (0.5%). This is indicative of the strict inclusion and exclusion criteria that are necessary to maintain satisfactory survival and safety outcomes when utilizing CRS and HIPEC for the treatment of gastric cancer peritoneal metastases.

Application of Peritonectomy Procedures and Other Surgical Techniques during Cytoreductive Surgery for Peritoneal Metastases of Gastric Cancer Origin

Sugarbaker described the peritonectomy procedures in 1995 as a series of surgical techniques that allow the complete resection of tumor deposits on the peritoneum and affected abdominal organs [30]. Subsequently, he published further technical details regarding suggested equipment and practical concepts that allow the optimal application of these procedures [31-34].

Other authors have since expanded on these foundations bringing in new approaches or technical modifications that have further enriched the surgical armamentarium for facing more challenging manifestations or localizations of gastric cancer peritoneal metastases (Figure 7) [35-40].

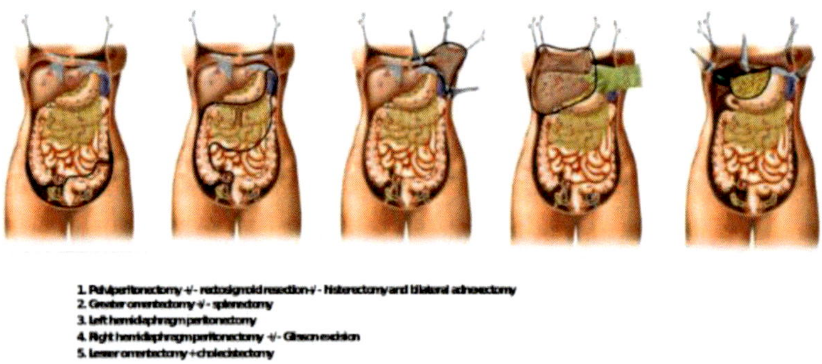

Figure 7. Modified Outline of Peritonectomy Procedures.

In the case of carcinomatosis of gastric cancer origin, cytoreductive surgery requires special strategies and adaptation of some of the classic peritonectomy procedure to allow a complete removal both of the primary tumor and its complex lymphatic network as well as the peritoneal metastases that sometime show particular aggressiveness.

However, it is important to note that, when selection criteria are correctly applied, the parietal peritonectomy procedures are generally limited to a few regions and the number of visceral resections outside of the primary tumor is also limited or not present. This means that the extent of the cytoreduction is generally less than in other pathologies and may therefore be more amenable to minimally invasive approaches, especially in cases of gastric cancer with positive peritoneal cytology only. However, the goal of achieving a complete macroscopic resection of the peritoneal disease and an oncologically appropriate resection of the primary tumor has to remain the same regardless of the surgical approach and it is a necessary condition for applying HIPEC in conjunction with CRS.

The most commonly required peritonectomy procedures and visceral resections performed during CRS for gastric cancer are the following:

Anterior Parietal (Epigastric) Peritonectomy and Resection of Previous Incision Sites

Patients undergoing CRS and HIPEC for gastric cancer have undergone one or two previous laparoscopy procedures and the excision of previous trocar sites is recommended. To facilitate it, it is advisable to place trocars in the midline when performing diagnostic laparoscopy for gastric cancer. When the trocars are placed in the midline, the sites can easily be excised with the midline incision performed to access the abdomen during CRS.

Together with the removal of the subcutaneous tissue and corresponding fascia, the excision involves the umbilicus and extends to the anterolateral epigastric peritoneum, the associated fat pad, the xyphoid process (to facilitate access to the subdiaphragmatic region and the hiatus) and the round and falciform ligaments of the liver.

Trocar scars from previous surgeries located outside the midline incision should be excised separately through all layers of the abdominal wall and should be left open to allow access of the chemotherapy solution during HIPEC (see Video 1).

Anterolateral Peritonectomy, Greater Omentectomy and Radical Gastrectomy With or Without Splenectomy

The anterolateral peritonectomy is complemented by and extended to include the greater omentum, the anterior leaf of the transverse colon mesentery, the peritoneum of the right paracolic sulcus (including the appendix) and the peritoneum of the subhepatic space.

The stripping of the anterior leaf of the transverse colon mesentery is started by dissecting the greater omentum off the transverse colon. Dissection in this plane is continued until the inferior border (or anterior surface) of the pancreas. In cases where a splenectomy is not indicated, it is important to remove the greater omentum completely, close to the splenic hilum to ensure the removal of potential small tumor deposits that can be present in this area.

In case of a splenectomy (without the need for a complete stripping of the left hemidiaphragm), the posterior peritoneal recess behind the spleen should be included in the resection, because a complete assessment of this space is difficult to perform visually or by palpation. The ligation and transection of the splenic vessels should be performed distally to avoid potential injury or ischemia to the distal portion of the pancreatic tail, which may lead to postoperative collections or a pancreatic fistula.

The peritonectomy procedures and visceral resections described above can be done en bloc as a single specimen. In our center, we prefer to perform this en bloc resection together with the radical gastrectomy and lymphadenectomy of the primary tumor removing the tissues as a single specimen (see Video 1).

Right diaphragmatic peritonectomy should only be done in case of multiple or diffuse nodules while isolated deposits can be resected individually, maintaining the integrity of the muscle or, in case of adherence or penetration, removing some muscle fibers. Nodules located on the peritoneum overlying the tendinous central portion of diaphragm can be more difficult to resect without opening the diaphragm. It is unknown if opening the diaphragm in these cases has negative oncologic implications.

Stripping of the Omental Bursa

The anatomical areas of the lesser sac are prone to involvement by gastric cancer peritoneal metastases, particularly when the primary tumor involves the posterior wall of the stomach. The peritoneal surfaces covering the anatomical boundaries of this space are: the posterior wall of the stomach, the peritoneal surface of the transverse mesocolon, the peritoneum overlying the anterior surface of the pancreas, the lesser omentum, the posterior boundary of the space behind the lesser omentum, the gallbladder and the peritoneum over the liver hilum. All of these peritoneal surfaces should be removed during CRS for gastric cancer. The hepatogastric ligament should be divided at its insertion into the liver extending upwards until the right diaphragmatic crus and the lesser omentum removed together with the gallbladder and the peritoneum overlying the hepatoduodenal ligament. The posterior peritoneal boundaries (floor of the omental bursa) are removed en bloc with the gastrectomy and lymphadenectomy specimen (see Video 1 and 2).

Gastrectomy and Lymphadenectomy

While HIPEC is used to address possible residual microscopic disease on the peritoneum, it is not able to affect the lymphatic spread of gastric cancer. It is therefore imperative to appropriately surgically address the possible lymphatic routes of spread by performing a complete lymphadenectomy according to the location of the tumor within the stomach.

The type of gastric resection is dictated by the size and location of the tumor, the lymphatic involvement, the histologic subtype and the presence of direct extension of the tumor into adjacent structures.

Regardless of the histologic subtype, the proximal transection line of the gastric specimen should be at least 5 cm from the tumor. The duodenal transection line should be at least 2 cm distal to the tumor. It is

resection of any tumor deposits of the small bowel is of paramount importance for a successful cytoreduction, especially because early tumor progression in this area would have a negative impact on the quality of life and symptom-free survival of patients. For this reason, the assessment of small bowel involvement and its resectability is an essential initial step prior to beginning any other resections in cytoreductive surgery for gastric cancer. If complete clearance of any visible tumor from the small bowel is not technically feasible, the procedure should be aborted and no attempts at partial cytoreduction should be done.

Isolated serosal nodules are removed sharply with scissors, either with a partial thickness resection when the mucosa is not affected or with a full-thickness wedge resection if involvement is deep. Full thickness defects are closed prior to HIPEC administration while partial thickness ones should remain open to allow better exposure to intraperitoneal chemotherapy. They should be oversewn with seromuscular sutures after completion of HIPEC.

The presence of a larger tumor deposit or a confluence of small deposits involving a segment of bowel, dictates the need for a segmental resection with primary anastomosis.

Special attention should be given to nodules situated at the border of the serosa and the mesentery. Excision with scissors should be done carefully, making sure sufficient blood supply is preserved and avoiding excessive use of cautery for hemostasis. It is also important to oversew these partial thickness defects carefully with interrupted sutures. Excision at these sites of the small bowel should be considered particularly high risk for fistula formation.

The presence of extensive small bowel involvement that would require multiple segmental resections or the presence of a retracted mesentery represents a contraindication to cytoreduction in gastric cancer carcinomatosis.

Segmental Ureter Resection and Reconstruction

Invasive tumor deposits in the pelvis can affect the ureter. The need for a segmental resection and primary anastomosis or other type of reconstruction of the ureter does not constitute per se a contraindication for cytoreduction of gastric cancer peritoneal metastases because neither the survival rate nor the complication rates seem to be directly correlated with ureteral resection (see Video 4).

If a resection and reconstruction of the ureter is performed, a ureteral catheter is left in place for at least 2 weeks. However, we do not place routine preoperative urinary catheters with the aim of identification of the ureters for cytoreductive surgery.

Salpingo-Oophorectomy

In women the ovaries can be the first, and occasionally, only site of peritoneal spread of gastric cancer (Krukenberg's tumors).

Metastatic involvement of the ovary, even though it clinically may appear as unilateral, should be treated with bilateral oophorectomy (see Video 2).

Gastrointestinal Reconstruction After Gastrectomy

Bowel reconstruction timing during CRS + HIPEC has been controversial. Classically, the optimal timing for any reconstruction or repair of digestive (and/or urinary) tract was considered to be after HIPEC with the aim of exposing the anastomotic ends to chemotherapys and reducing the risk of recurrence at the suture line.

The negative effects of high concentrations of regional chemotherapy on the tissue healing process is well known [41, 42], as is the administration of anti-vascular endothelial growth factor monoclonal antibodies [43, 44].

Furthermore, after HIPEC, anastomoses safety can be compromised by intestinal edema generated by HIPEC itself and the surgical time addition required for its assembly and administration. Intestinal wall thickness determines the adequacy of mechanical stapling height and the adjustment of manual knotting to avoid ischemia and tissue tear.

We prefer to always perform digestive tract reconstruction before HIPEC administration [45] with special care to confirm complete absence of tumor at the ends to be anastomosed (see Video 2). Only the approximation of serosal edges resulting from partial thickness tumor nodule resection is performed after HIPEC (see Video 4).

HIPEC administration after digestive anastomoses performance during closed HIPEC modality confirms the efficacy of this strategy and, most likely, influences anastomotic safety.

Once all of the procedures required for complete cytoreduction are complete, the type of reconstruction will depend on the kind of gastrectomy performed. There are a variety of described reconstruction options but the most widely utilized is the Roux-en-Y reconstruction for both total and subtotal gastrectomy while the classic (see Video 1 and 2)

Post gastrectomy reconstruction options of Billroth I and Billroth II are rarely appropriate for cytoreductive surgery. In this chapter, we will describe the reconstruction options we have used most frequently in our center and some relevant technical details important to improve the safety of the reconstruction.

We take special care in the preparation of the distal esophageal transection line in order to optimize the safety of the esophago-jejunal suture line. The muscular layer is divided circumferentially leaving the mucosal layer approximately 1 cm longer in order to ensure optimal closure of the mucosal layer around the anvil of the EEA stapler (Figure 8).

In patients who have had prior partial gastrectomy and either a Billroth II or Roux-en-Y reconstruction, we utilize a Roux-en-Y esophago- or gastrojejunostomy for reconstruction after CRS and HIPEC. In patients without prior gastrectomy who require a total gastrectomy during CRS and HIPEC, our preferred reconstruction technique has been with an interposed isoperistaltic jejunal loop (of approximately 40 cm) anastomosed to the esophagus and the duodenum (Figure 9 and Video 3). The esophago-jejunostomy in this type of reconstruction can be performed in an end-to-end or an end-to-side fashion.

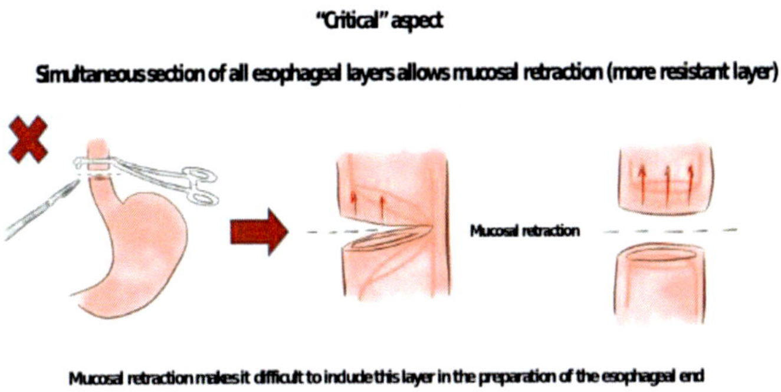

a

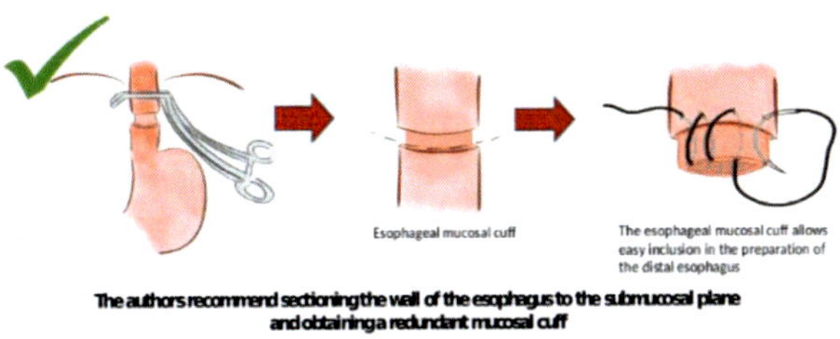

b

Figure 8. Preparation of the Esophageal end to facilitate a safe esophageal-jejunal anastomosis.

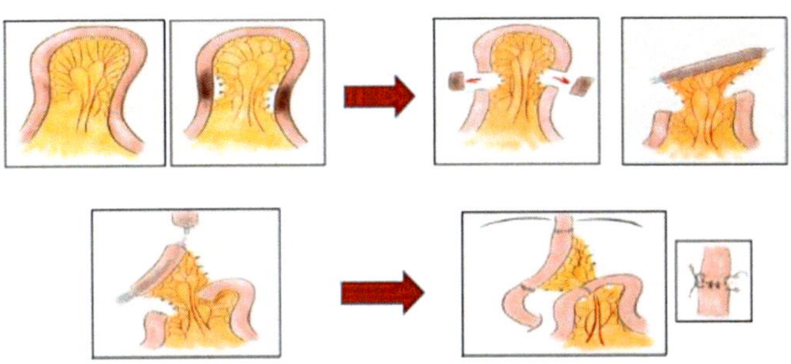

Figure 9. Technical modality used by the authors for duodeno- esophageal reconstruction using an isolated jejunal segment interposition (Longmire).

Once the EEA mechanical anastomosis is created, it is reinforced with seromuscular interrupted sutures circumferentially and the anastomosis tested intraoperatively.

The distal end of the interposed segment is then anastomosed to the duodenum with a hand-sewn end-to-end anastomosis. The ends of the small bowel at the site of the resection of the interposition segment are anastomosed in the same fashion.

We give great importance to irrigation and aspiration of abundant amounts of physiological saline in the abdominal cavity repeatedly during many moments of CRS with the aim of eliminating the largest possible amount of FCCs and avoiding the entrapment of remaining ones in detached areas prior to HIPEC, based on the knowledge of peritoneal seeding pathophysiology (see Video 1,2 and 3). Results of Kuramoto's [46] work go in this direction, although a recent multicenter randomized study from the EXPEL group doesn´t confirm a survival advantage of this procedure [47].

Postoperative Complications after Cytoreductive Surgery for Gastric Cancer Peritoneal Metastases

Patients with gastric cancer peritoneal metastases have a high rate of preoperative malnutrition, present in 62-83% of the cases [48].

Malnutrition is associated with a higher rate of postoperative complications, a slower rate of postoperative recovery, lower quality of life and decreased survival [49-50].

Basic nutritional assessment should be done in all patients who are potential candidates for CRS and HIPEC for gastric cancer while a more detailed and specialized evaluation is necessary in patients with a clinical suspicion of malnutrition. Postoperative nutritional follow up should be continued for at least 1 year after surgery [51-52].

Complications after CRS and HIPEC can be a direct result of the cytoreductive surgery, related to the intraperitoneal chemotherapy, the hyperthermia or caused by a combination of factors. Surgical complications are the most important and frequent cause of significant complications and may cause a delay or impossibility of further oncological treatment for patients.

There are many classification systems for postoperative complications but not one of them has been identified as optimal for use in CRS and HIPEC. Elias, in 1994, described a classification system adapted for use in CRS and HIPEC specifically with 6 grades of complications. Grade 0: no complications; Grade 1: complications that do not require treatment or require only minor interventions such as oral antibiotics or basic laboratory checks; Grade 2: complications that require moderate interventions such as intravenous medications, parenteral nutrition, prolonged nasogastric suctioning, placement of a pleural catheter; Grade 3: complications that require readmission to the hospital, surgical intervention or an interventional radiology procedure; Grade 4: complications that lead to chronic sequelae, require organ resection or creation of ostomy and Grade 5: complications that lead to death [53].

In the 5th Biannual Peritoneal Surface Oncology Workshop in Milan in 2006 a consensus was reached recommending the utilization of the *Commom Terminology Criteria for Adverse Events* (CTCAE) classification system for the evaluation of complications following CRS and HIPEC. It is an extensive classification system that categorizes 310 types of complications divided in to 28 categories, evaluating anatomically based complications as well as patophysiologic derangement and is therefore useful for CRS and HIPEC because it can capture both surgical as well as chemotherapy-related complications [54].

The rate of Grade II, III and IV complications after CRS and HIPEC is between 30- 65%. Surgical complications can reach 30% and predominantly include anastomotic complications, fistulas, abdominal collections and abscess as well as postoperative bleeding. They lead to a reoperation rate of approximately 10% [55, 56]. Investigators from the Washington Hospital Center, one of the leading centers for CRS in the world, found that the rate of severe postoperative complications is related to the extent of the peritoneal disease measured by the Peritoneal Cancer Index, the duration of surgery and the number of intestinal anastomoses [57].

Although the rate of major complications in CRS and HIPEC is generally similar to the rate of complications in other major surgical procedures, the postoperative management should be especially careful and able to detect and respond to any early signs of complications considering that the patients undergoing CRS and HIPEC are more fragile due to their extensive oncological treatments.

Although surgical complications after CRS and HIPEC are similar to complications that occur after conventional abdominal surgery, they can be masked or worsened by the effects of the HIPEC chemotherapy which can be systemic, most often gastrointestinal or hematologic. The peritonectomy procedures themselves, possibly augmented by the effects of intraperitoneal chemotherapy can cause a loss of the clinical signs of peritoneal irritation and make early clinical diagnosis of abdominal complications more difficult. The immediate postoperative recovery after CRS and HIPEC should be performed by appropriately trained personnel and in an environment that allows close monitoring, usually in an intensive care unit. In case of clinical suspicion of a complication, there should be a low threshold for performing the appropriate laboratory or radiological tests with the aim of early diagnosis and a greater chance of resolution with non-invasive or less-invasive means avoiding surgical re-interventions.

The published mortality rates after CRS and HIPEC ranges from 0-14%. The majority of published series report a mortality rate of 2-6%. The mortality rates are influenced by the origin of the carcinomatosis and the associated aggressiveness of the CRS and HIPEC procedure in particular by the PCI, the number of peritonectomy procedures and anastomoses and the transfusion rate. Patients with pseudomyxoma peritonei, because of the associated high volume of peritoneal disease, generally show the highest rates of postoperative mortality.

The most common causes of mortality after CRS and HIPEC are gastrointestinal surgical complications (anastomotic leak and perforation), bone marrow insufficency, respiratory insufficiency, pulmonary embolus and methicillin-resistant Staphylococcus aureus infections. Various factors have been shown to be predictors of mortality after CRS and HIPEC including the presence of high volume ascites, low performance status and preoperative bowel obstruction [58, 59].

The incidence of postoperative morbidity and mortality after CRS and HIPEC is related to the experience of the surgical team. Several studies have evaluated the learning curve for CRS and HIPEC. It is also evident that studies with >100 reported cases have lower reported incidence of morbidity and mortality [60, 61]. It is also important to consider the relationship of postoperative morbidity, a reflection of the quality of surgical care, with the ability to complete further necessary oncological treatments. A significant delay in the administration of planned adjuvant treatment or the inability to deliver it will have direct negative repercussions on the overall oncological outcome [62].

The organizational and technical structure of a team or medical facility has a direct influence on the ultimate outcome of postoperative complications and can be expressed through the *failure-to-rescue* (FTR) rate. FTR can therefore serve as a measure of the impact of institutional and team characteristics on outcomes independent of other patient or disease-related factors [63, 64].

Overall, optimization of patient selection criteria and an increased experience in peritoneal surface malignancy surgery has lead to a decrease in rates of complications of CRS and HIPEC over time [63].

The Role of Minimally Invasive Surgery (MIS) in the Surgical Treatment of Gastric Cancer Peritoneal Metastases

The standard approach for CRS and HIPEC for treatment of peritoneal metastases regardless of origin is open surgery. This is often determined by the volume of peritoneal disease and the need for extensive and multiple peritonectomy procedures which are not suitable for a minimally invasive approach.

However, over the last few years, there has been emerging evidence to support the use of minimally invasive techniques to perform CRS in select cases of very low peritoneal tumor burden [65].

Considering the fact that gastric cancer tumor biology requires very strict inclusion criteria for CRS and HIPEC, often limited to patients with radiologically occult minimal peritoneal disease or those with positive cytology only, the applicability of MIS may be greater than in other types of peritoneal metastases.

However, the published experience utilizing minimally invasive surgery in patients with gastric cancer carcinomatosis so far is limited to the feasibility of laparoscopic HIPEC (without cytoreduction) in patients with limited peritoneal metastases. In 2017, Badgewell et al. performed a Phase II study of iterative laparoscopic HIPEC with mitomycin C and cisplatin among 19 patients of which 5 achieved resolution of peritoneal disease (by cytology and biopsy) and proceeded to standard gastrectomy. The complication rate for HIPEC was 11% (4 of 38 procedures) and the 30-day mortality rate was 0% [66]. The same group expanded their experience publishing the results of 20 patients undergoing gastrectomy with CRS and HIPEC (open surgery) after prior laparoscopic HIPEC used as neoadjuvant treatment. Median OS from the date of diagnosis of metastatic disease was 24.2 months; and median OS from the date of cytoreduction, gastrectomy, and HIPEC was 16.1 months [67].

In our center, we have begun applying minimally invasive (laparoscopic) gastrectomy and lymphadenectomy combined with laparoscopic HIPEC for patients with gastric cancer and positive peritoneal cytology in 2019. A standard laparoscopic complete omentectomy, gastrectomy (subtotal or total) and D2 or D1plus lymphadenectomy is performed. We use a small periumbilical incision as extraction of the specimen in order to allow a thorough examination of the small bowel by palpation to detect any tumor deposits at the border of the bowel and mesentery that can be difficult to detect visually but can easily be performed using the same small periumbilical incision. Reconstruction is performed with stapled intracorporeal Roux-en-Y esophago- or gastrojejunostomy. Following resection and reconstruction, laparoscopic HIPEC is performed placing the inflow and outflow catheters through the existing trocar sites. Preliminary results in 5 patients show that the procedure is feasible and safe with no anastomotic leak and 1 grade II postoperative complication.

The Moises Broggi Hospital Experience (Peritoneal Carcinomatosis Program of Catalonia) of CRS and HIPEC for Gasric Cáncer

All data regarding the activities of the center have been maintained in a dedicated prospective database.

The database contains records of 1300 patients with various types of surgically treated PM performed from August 2006 to August 2020 of which 58 (5%) had gastric PM.

Patients with a performance status of 0-2, limited peritoneal metastases defined as peritoneal cancer index (PCI) of <12, a resectable primary tumor and no other sites of distant metastases are considered potential candidates. The standard clinical pathways includes diagnostic laparoscopy, systemic chemotherapy for 4 cycles, repeat diagnostic laparoscopy prior to gastrectomy, CRS and HIPEC.

HIPEC consists of CDDP 80 mg/m2 + Doxorrubicin 15 mg/m2, at 42.1°C (median) for 60 minutes.

The exposed data were subjected to an external evaluation by the Agència de Qualitat I Avaluació Sanitàries de Catalunya (AQuAS).

There were 58 patients (34 females and 24 males) with a mean age of 52.6 years.

In 8 patients (13.8%) PM presented as recurrent disease after a prior gastrectomy while 50 (86.2%) had synchronous PM and underwent gastrectomy at the time of peritonectomy and HIPEC.

Sixteen patients had no macroscopic PM: 10 had positive washings by cytology and 6 by molecular analysis.

The mean number of affected regions were 3.5/13 and the mean PCI was 5.3/39.

Thc majority (47/58) had a total gastrectomy with D2 lymphadenectomy. Surgical procedures performed are summarized in Table 1.

Significant postoperative morbidity was low: ICU readmission in 1 (1.7%), hospital readmissions in 8 (13.5%) and urgent reoperation in 5 (8.6%) cases. The reason for urgent reoperation were 3 intestinal obstruction (no recurrence) cases, 2 intestinal fistula (1 anastomotic leak) and 1 hemoperitoneum.

Table 1. Surgical procedures

Surgical Procedures	Number of patients	%
Total gastrectomy	44	76%
Partial gastrectomy	6	10%
Previous gastrectomy	8	14%
Splenectomy	22	38%
Small bowel resection	11	19%
Rectosigmoid colon resection	4	7%
Right colectomy	5	9%
Transverse colectomy	7	13%
Left colectomy	4	7%
Partial bladder resection	2	3.4%
Ureteral resection	3	5.2%
Pelviperitonectomy	8	14%
Adnexectomy +/- cul-de-sac-ectomy	28	48%
Upper Quadrant Peritonectomy	8	13.8%

Mortality occurred in 1 pt. (1.7%) due to bronchoaspiration.

After a median follow up of 12.3 months 28 patients died (48.3%), 5 were alive with disease (8.6%) and 18 were disease-free (31.3%).

Median survival was 20.6 months (IC 95%: 13.9 – 27.2 months) for the whole group but varied significantly based on extent of peritoneal disease and histologic subtype.

The best survival (32.8 months median) was seen in patients with a PCI $\leq$ 11, complete resection (CC-0) and no "signet ring" histology.

List of Videos Attached to the Chapter on CRS Techniques in Gastric Cancer Associated with Peritoneal Metastases

Video 1: Gastric Cancer with Synchronous PM (Male Patient)

Surgical strategy: Total gastrectomy, lymphadenectomy associated to splenectomy, and transverse colectomy. Proximal small bowel resection.

Cul-de-sac-ectomy

Roux-en-Y reconstruction

Hand sewn colo-colic anastomosis

Video 2: Metachronic Gastric PM (Female Patient). Previous Gastrectomy

Preparing the patient for CRS + HIPEC

Surgical strategy: redo gastrectomy, cholecystectomy, omental bursectomy and splenectomy en bloc

Bilateral adnexectomy and cul-de-sac-ectomy

Resection of implants of the abdominal wall

Roux-en-Y reconstruction

Technical realization of the HIPEC (open "coliseum" technique)

Video 3: Gastric Cancer with Synchronous PM (Female Patient)

Surgical strategy: total gastrectomy and lymphadenectomy D2.

Resection of nodules from the sigmoid colon serosa

Esophago-duodenal reconstruction with jejunal interposition (Longmire)

Video 4: Iterative CRS+HIPEC in Recurrent Gastric PM

Surgical strategy: CRS of the lateral wall of the pelvis with segmental resection of the middle ureter

Reconstruction of the urinary tract with interposition of an isolated segment of the small bowel

Cytoreduction of the intestine and mesentery by intestinal segmental resection and excision of isolated serous implants

REFERENCES

[1] Hioki M, Gotohda N, Konishi M, et al. Predictive factors improving survival after gastrectomy in gastric cancer patients with peritoneal carcinomatosis. *World J Surg.* 2010;34:555-62.

[2] Leake PA, Cardoso R, Seevaratnam R et al. A systematic review of the accuracy and utility of peritoneal cytology in patients with gastric cancer. *Gastric Cancer.* 2012;15 Sup 1: S27-37.

[3] Wei J, Wu ND, Liu BR. Regional but fatal: Intraperitoneal metastasis in gastric cancer. *World J Gastroenterol.* 2016;22:7478-85.

[4] Thomassen I, van Gestel YR, van Ramshorst B et al. Peritoneal carcinomatosis of gastric origin: a population-based study on incidence, survival and risk factors. *Int J Cancer.* 2014;134:622-8.

[5] *TNM Classification of Malignant Tumours*. 7th ed. UICC; 2009.

[6] *NNCN Clinical Practice Guidelines in Gastric Cancer* V.2016. Available from: https://www.nccn.org/.

[7] Sano T, Aiko T. New Japanese classifications and treatment guidelines for gastric cancer: revision concepts and major revised points. *Gastric Cancer.* 2011;14(2):97-100.

[8] Wagner AD, Unverzagt S, Grothe W, et al. Chemotherapy for advanced gastric cancer. *Cochrane Database Syst Rev.* 2010;3:CD004064.

[9] Deng K, Zhu H, Chen M, et al. Prognostic Significance of Molecular Analysis of Peritoneal Fluid for Patients with Gastric Cancer: A

Meta-Analysis. *PLoS One.* 2016 Mar 17;11(3):e0151608. doi: 10.1371/journal.pone.0151608. eCollection 2016.

[10] Magge D, Zenatti M, Mavanur A, et al. Aggresive locoregional surgical therapy for gastric peritoneal carciomatosis. *Ann Surg Oncol.* 2014;21(5):1448-55.

[11] Verwaal J, van Tinteren H, van Ruth S, Zoetmulder FA. Predicting the survival of patients with peritoneal carcinomatosis of colorectal origin treated by aggressive cytoreduction and hyperthermic intraperitoneal chemotherapy. *Br J Surg.* 2004;91:739-46.

[12] Therasse P, Arbuck SG, Eisenhauer EA, et al. New guidelines to evaluate the response to treatment in solid tumors. European Organization for Research and Treatment of Cancer, National Cancer Institute of the United States, National Cancer Institute of Canada. *J Natl Cancer Inst.* 2000;92:205-16.

[13] Pomel C, Appleyard T, Gouy S, et al. The role of laparoscopy to evaluate candidates for complete cytoreduction of peritoneal carcinomatosis and hyperthermic intraperitoneal chemotherapy. *Eur J Surg Oncol.* 2005;31:540-3.

[14] Valle M, Garofalo A. Laparoscopic staging of peritoneal surface malignancies. *Eur J Surg Oncol.* 2006;32:625-7.

[15] Japanese Gastric Cancer Association. Japanese classification of gastric carcinoma: 3rd edition. *Gastric Cancer.* 2011;14:101-112.

[16] Iwamoto A. Intraoperative chemotherapy with intraperitoneal activated carbon particles adsorbing mitomycin C against peritoneal dissemination of gastric cancer. *Gan To Kagaku Ryoho.* 1989;16:2748-51.

[17] Fujimoto S. Improved mortality rate of gastic carcinoma patients with peritoneal carcinomatosis treated with intraperitoneal hyperthermic chemoperfusion combined with surgery. *Cancer.* 1997;79:884-91.

[18] Ouchi K. Therapeutic significance of palliative operations for gastric cancer for survival and quality of life. *J Surg Oncol.* 1998;69:41-4.

[19] Gilly FN. Regional chemotherapy (with mitomycin C) and intra-operative hyperthermia for digestive cancers with peritoneal carcinomatosis. *Hepatogastroenterology.* 1994;41:124-9.

[20] Ronnett BM. Disseminated peritoneal adenomucinosis and peritoneal mucinous carcinomatosis. A clinicopathologic analysis of 109 cases with emphasis on distinguishing pathologic features, site of origin, prognosis, and relationship to "pseudomyxoma peritonei." *Am J Surg Pathol.* 1995;19:1390-408.

[21] Zoetmulder FAN, Verwaal V. Hyperthermic intraperitoneal chemotherapy (HIPEC) with mitomycin C significantly improves survival in patients with peritoneal carcinomatosis of colorectal origin (abstract). *ASCO Prog Proc.* 2002;21:147a.

[22] Jacquet P, Sugarbaker PH. Clinical research methodologies in diagnosis and staging of patients with peritoneal carcinomatosis. *Cancer Treat Res.* 1996;82:359-74.

[23] Gomez Portilla A, Sugarbaker PH, Chang D. Second-look surgery after cytoreduction and intraperitoneal chemotherapy for peritoneal carcinomatosis from colorectal cancer: analysis of prognostic features. *World J Surg.* 1999;23:23-9.

[24] Berthet B, Sugarbaker TA, Chang D, Sugarbaker PH. Quantitative methodologies for selection of patients with recurrent abdominopelvic sarcoma for treatment. *Eur J Cancer.* 1999;35:413-9.

[25] Glehen O, Gilly FN, Arvieux C, et al. Peritoneal carcinomatosis from gastric cancer: a multi-institutional study of 159 patients treated by cytoreductive surgery combined with perioperative intraperitoneal chemotherapy. *Ann Surg Oncol.* 2010;17:2370-7.

[26] Yonemura Y, Kawamura T, Bandou E, et al. Treatment of peritoneal dissemination from gastric cancer by peritonectomy and chemohyperthermic peritoneal perfusion. *Br J Surg.* 2005;92:370-5.

[27] Hall JJ, Loggie BW, Shen P, et al. *J Gastrointestinal Surg.* 2004;8:454-63.

[28] Smeenk RM, Verwaal VJ, Zoetmulder FA. Learning curve of combined modality treatment in peritoneal surface disease. *Br J Surg.* 2007;94:1408-14.

[29] Yann TD, Links M, Fransi S, et al. Learning curve for cytoreductive surgery and perioperative intraperitoneal chemotherapy for peritoneal surface malignancy – a journey to becoming a National Funded Peritonectomy Center. *Ann Surg Oncol.* 2007;14:2270-80.

[30] Sugarbaker PH. Peritonectomy procedures. *Ann Surg.* 1995;221:29-42.

[31] Sugarbaker PH. Peritoneal Carcinomatosis. *Principles of Management.* Boston: Kluwer; 1996.

[32] Sugarbaker PH. Peritonectomy procedures. *Surg Oncol Clin N Am.* 2003;12:703-27.

[33] Sugarbaker PH. Peritonectomy using electrosurgery with a ball tip on high voltaje and pure cut. In: *Electrosurgery: Principles, Fundamentals and Benefits.* NOVA Science Publishers, NY; 2017.

[34] Sugarbaker PH. Circumferential cutaneous traction for exposure of the layers of the abdominal wall. *J Surg Oncol.* 2008;98:472-5.

[35] Yonemura Y, Fujimura T, Fushida S, et al. Peritonectomy as a treatment modality for patients with peritoneal dissemination from gastric cancer. In: Nakashima T, Yamaguchy T, editors. *Multimodality Theraphy for Gastric Cancer.* Tokyo: Spring-Verlag; 1999. P. 71-80.

[36] Yonemura Y, Fujimura T, Fushida S, et al. Techniques of peritonectomy for advanced and recurrent gastric cancer with peritoneal dissemination. In Siewert JR, Roder JD, editors. 2 nd *International Gastric Cancer Congress.* Bologna: Monduzzi; 1997. P. 1365-9.

[37] Yonemura Y, Fujimura T, Fushida S, et al. A new surgical approah (peritonectomy) for the treatment of peritoneal dissemination. *Hepatogastroenterology.* 1999; 46:601-9.

[38] Bijelic L, Sugarbaker PH. Cytoreduction of the small bowel surfaces. *J Surg Oncol.* 2008;97:176-9.

[39] Deraco M, Baratti D, Kusamura S, et al. Surgical tecnique of parietal and visceral peritonectomy for peritoneal surface malignancies. *J Surg Oncol.* 2009;100:321-8.

[40] Barrios P, Ramos, I, Crusellas O, Sabia D, Mompart S and Martín-Baranera M. Colorectal anastomosis during cytoreductive radical surgery in patients with peritoneal surface malignancies. Validation of a new technique (without stoma) to prevent anastomosis leakage in more tan 1000 procedures. *Clinical and Translational Oncology.* 2021. https://doi.org/10.1007/s12094-020-02511-7.

[41] Sugarbaker PH. New standard of care for appendiceal epitelial neoplasms and pseudomixoma peritonei sindrome? *Lancet Oncol.* 2006; 7(1):69-76.

[42] Casado-Adam A, Alderman R, Stuart OA, Chang D, Sugarbaker PH. Gastrointestinal complications in 147 consecutive patients with peritoneal surface malignancy treated by cytoreductive surgery and perioperative intraperitoneal chemotherapy. *Int J Surg Oncol.* 2011:468698. Doi: 10.1155/2011/468698. Epub 2011 Oct 16.

[43] Heinzeeling JH, Huerta S. Bowel perforation from bevacizumab for the Treatment of metastasic colon cáncer: incidence, etiology and management. *Curr Surg.* 2006;63:334-437.

[44] Saif MW, Elfiky A, Salem RR. Gastrointestinal perforation due bevacizumab in colorectal cancer. *Ann Surg Oncol.* 2007;14:1860-1869.

[45] Barrios P, Ramos I, Escayola C, Martín-Baranera M. *Implementación y desarrollo de un programa de tratamiento de la carcinomatosis peritoneal en Cataluña. Indicaciones y resultados clínicos con la técnica de Sugarbaker.* Barcelona: Agència d'Avaluació de Tecnologia i Recerca Mèdiques. Servei Català de la Salut. Departament de Salut. Generalitat de Catalunya; 2009. [*Implementation and development of a peritoneal carcinomatosis treatment program in Catalonia. Indications and clinical results with the Sugarbaker technique.* Barcelona: Agency for the Evaluation of Medical Technology and Research. Catalan Health Service. Department of Health. Government of Catalonia]

[46] Kuramoto M, Shimada S, Ikeshima S, et al. Extensive intraoperative peritoneal lavage as a standard prophylactic strategy for peritoneal recurrence in patients with gastric carcinoma. *Ann Surg.* 2009;250(2):242-6.

[47] Yang HK, Ji J, Han SU, et al. EXPEL study group. Extensive peritoneal lavage with saline after curative gastrectomy for gastric cancer (EXPEL): a multicenter randomized controlled trial. *Lancet Gastroenterol Hepatol.* 2020 Nov 27;S2468-1253(20)30315-0.

[48] Andreyev HJ, Norman AR, Oates J, et al. Why do patients with weight loss have a worse outcome when undergoing chemotherapy for gastrointestinal malignancies? *Eur J Cancer.* 1998;34:503-9.

[49] Mullen JL, Buzby GB, Waldman MT, et al. Prediction of operative morbidity and mortality by preoperative nutritional assessment. *Surg Forum.* 1979;30:80-2.

[50] Andreyev HJ, Norman AR, Oates J, et al. Why do patients with weight loss have a worse outcome when undergoing chemotherapy for gastrointestinal malignancies? *Eur J Cancer.* 1998;34:503-9.

[51] Huhmann MB, Cunningham RS. Importance of nutritional screening in the treatment of cancer- related weight loss. *Lancet Oncol.* 2005;6:334-43.

[52] Kondrup J, Allison SP, Elia M, et al. Educational and Clinical Practice Committee, European Society of Parenteral and Enteral Nutrition (ESPEN). ESPEN guidelines for nutrition screening 2002. *Clin Nutr.* 2003;22:415-21.

[53] Elias D, Detroz B, Debaene B, et al. Treatment of peritoneal carcinomatosis by intraperitoneal chemo-hyperthermia: reliable and unreliable concepts. *Hepatogastroenterology.* 1994;41:207-13.

[54] *Common Terminology Criteria for Adverse Events (CTCAE)* versión 3.0.

[55] Butterworth SA, Panton ON, Klaassen DJ, et al. Morbility and mortality associated with peritoneal chemotherapy for pseudomyxoma peritonei. *Am J Surg.* 2002;183:529-32.

[56] Smeenk R, Verwaal VJ, Zoetmulder FA. Toxicity and mortality of cytoreduction and intraoperative hyperthermic chemotherapy in

pseudomyxoma peritonei: report of 103 procedures. *Eur J Surg Oncol.* 2006;32(2):186-90.

[57] Stephens AD, Alderman R, Chang D, et al. Morbility and mortality analysis of 200 treatments with cytoreductive surgery and hyperthermic intraoperative intraperitoneal chemotherapy using coliseum technique. *Ann Surg Oncol.* 1999;6:790-6.

[58] Elias DM, Pocard M. Treatment and prevention of peritoneal carcinomatosis from colorectal cancer. *Surg Oncol Clin N Am.* 2003;12:543-59.

[59] Shen P, Levine EA, Hall J, et al. Factors predicting survival after intraperitoneal hyperthermic chemotherapy with mitomycin C after cytoreductive surgery for patients with peritoneal carcinomatosis. *Arch Surg*. 2003;138:26-33.

[60] Sugarbaker PH, Alderman R, Edwards G, et al. Prospective morbidity and mortality assessment of citoreductive surgery plus perioperative intraperitoneal chemotherapy to treat peritoneal dissemination of appendiceal mucinous malignancy. *Ann Surg Oncol.* 2006;13(5):635-44.

[61] Aloia TA, Zimmitti G, Conrad C, et al. Return to intended oncologic treatment: a novel metric for evaluating the quality of oncosurgical therapy for malignancy. *J Surg Oncol.* 2014;110:107-14.

[62] Ghaferi AA, Birkmeyer JD, Dimick JB. Complications, failure-to-rescue, and mortality with major inpatient surgery in medicare patients. *Ann Surg.* 2009;250:1029-34.

[63] Massarweh NN, Anaya DA, Kougias P, et al. Variation and impact of multiple complications on failure to rescue after inpatient surgery. *Ann Surg.* 2017;266:59-65.

[64] Barlett EK, Meise Ch, Roses RF, et al. Morbidity and Mortality of Cytorreduction with Intra- peritoneal Chemotherapy: Outcomes from the ACS NSQIP Database. *Ann Surg Oncol.* 2014;21:1494-500.

[65] Arjona-Sanchez A, Aziz O, Passot Ga et al. Laparoscopic cytoreductive surgery and hyperthermic intraperitoneal chemotherapy for limited peritoneal metastasis. The PSOGI

international collaborative registry. *EJSO* 2020; https://doi.org/10.106/j.ejso.2020.11.140.

[66] Badgwell B, Blum M, Das Prajnan, et al. Phase II Trial of Laparoscopic Hyperthermic Intraperitoneal Chemoperfusion for Peritoneal Carcinomatosis or Positive Peritoneal Cytology in Patients with Gastric Adenocarcinoma. *Ann Surg Oncol.* 2017;24:3338–44.

[67] Badgwell B, Ikoma N, Murphy MB, et al. A Phase II Trial of Cytoreduction, Gastrectomy, and Hyperthermic Intraperitoneal Perfusion with Chemotherapy for Patients with Gastric Cancer and Carcinomatosis or Positive Cytology. *Ann Surg Oncol.* 2021;28(1):258-64. https://doi.org/10.1245/s10434-020-08739-5.

In: Gastric Peritoneal Carcinomatosis
Editors: F. López Mozos et al.
ISBN: 978-1-53619-487-6

Chapter 8

ROLE OF INTRAPERITONEAL CHEMOTHERAPY IN GASTRIC CANCER

Israel Manzanedo, PhD and Fernando Pereira*, PhD
Hospital Universitario de Fuenlabrada, Madrid, Spain

ABSTRACT

Gastric cancer (GC) is the third cause of cancer-related deaths in the world, with less than 25% survivors at 5 years. These results are related to the high incidence of peritoneal metastases (PM) in these patients. Nowadays, the standard treatment for GC with PM is palliative systemic chemotherapy (SCT) with a median survival of 6 months.

From the 2000s, the treatment with cytoreductive surgery (CRS) and Hyperthermic Intraperitoneal Chemotherapy (HIPEC) has been gaining popularity for different neoplastic diseases that involve the peritoneal surface. With this treatment, the surgeon can remove all macroscopic disease, but the residual microscopic disease is the most probable cause of future relapses. The use of HIPEC tries to eliminate this microscopic disease through high cytostatic doses acting locally, with the synergy and the effect of heat. The use of CRS and HIPEC has been studied for GC with PM, with promising results in selected patients, obtaining survival

* Corresponding Author's E-mail: fernando.pereira@salud.madrid.org.

rates never seen before. Also, Early Postoperative Intraperitoneal Chemotherapy (EPIC) can be added to CRS and HIPEC in patients with good performance status in experienced centers, improving the results.

Moreover, HIPEC and other intraperitoneal chemotherapy techniques have been used to prevent peritoneal recurrences in patients diagnosed on locally advanced GC without macroscopic PM (adjuvant or prophylactic HIPEC).

Even, intraperitoneal chemotherapy (laparoscopic HIPEC and neoadjuvant intraperitoneal and systemic chemotherapy -NIPS-) has been used as neoadjuvant treatment to reduce peritoneal disease burden in order to improve the rate of patients in whom complete cytoreduction can be achieved.

INTRODUCTION

Gastric cancer (GC) is the third cause of cancer-related deaths in the world, with a 5-year overall survival (OS) less than 25%. The high incidence of peritoneal metastases (PM) contributes greatly to this dismal prognosis. Nowadays, the standard treatment for GC with PM is palliative systemic chemotherapy (SCT) with a median survival of 6 months, even for the patients with isolated positive peritoneal cytology (microscopic PM), in absence of macroscopic nodules, which are classified as M1 and have similar prognosis to those with macroscopic PM.

From the 2000s, the treatment with cytoreductive surgery (CRS) and Hyperthermic IntraPEritoneal Chemotherapy (HIPEC) has been gaining popularity for different neoplastic diseases that involve the peritoneal surface. With this combined treatment, the surgeon can remove all macroscopic disease, and HIPEC tries to eliminate the residual microscopic disease, which is though as a highly probable cause of future relapses at the peritoneal surface. HIPEC works through high cytostatic doses acting locally, with the synergy and the effect of heat. The use of CRS and HIPEC has been studied for GC with PM with promising results in selected patients, obtaining survival rates never seen before. Also, Early Postoperative Intraperitoneal Chemotherapy (EPIC) has been used in addition to CRS and HIPEC trying to improve the oncological outcome.

Otherwise, adjuvant of prophylactic HIPEC and other intraperitoneal chemotherapy techniques have been used to prevent peritoneal recurrences in patients diagnosed on locally advanced GC without macroscopic PM.

Even, intraperitoneal chemotherapy has been used as neoadjuvant treatment to reduce peritoneal disease burden in order to improve the rate of patients in whom complete cytoreduction can be achieved (laparoscopic HIPEC and neoadjuvant intraperitoneal and systemic chemotherapy -NIPS-).

Finally, patients with high volume peritoneal disease can be treated by palliative intraperitoneal chemotherapy to control the symptoms resulting from malignant ascites, using laparoscopic HIPEC or pressurized intraperitoneal aerosol chemotherapy (PIPAC).

This chapter aims to update the management of the different applications of intraperitoneal chemotherapy for GC, based on the literature and the experience of the authors.

Rationale for Intraperitoneal Chemotherapy in GC

Intraperitoneal chemotherapy is the local administration of antitumoral drugs inside the peritoneal cavity. This regional application allows the direct infusion of chemotherapy at high doses in the peritoneum. The peritoneal-plasma barrier (PPB) is the reason for the poor success of SCT for the treatment of peritoneal implants because it does not allow the drug to pass from the blood to the peritoneum. Moreover, if the drug is administered into the peritoneal cavity, the PPB will not allow it to penetrate in the bloodstream, at least partially; therefore, we can achieve high local drug concentration without the side effects derived from its systemic administration. With intraperitoneal infusion of the chemotherapy, the time and dose of exposure of PM is increased with minimal systemic toxic effects [1]. However, the effectiveness of anticancer drugs depends on the direct contact of the chemotherapy solution with the cancer nodule, and, furthermore, it is known that the penetration of the drug into the tissues is limited to a few cell layers or a few millimeters, so that a complete cytoreduction is essential to ensure the correct action of chemotherapy [2, 3].

There are different options for intraperitoneal chemotherapy [1, 3]. Currently, the intraoperative administration is the most frequent. HIPEC is usually administered after surgical removal of macroscopic PM through CRS. HIPEC can be administered by laparoscopy (LHIPEC) in three clinical scenarios: 1) after laparoscopic CRS in those cases where this is possible; 2) as neoadjuvant therapy to reduce the peritoneal disease burden in order to enhance the number of patients in whom complete cytoreduction can be achieved; and 3) as palliative treatment in patients with unresectable PM to improve their quality of life controlling their symptoms. Intraperitoneal chemotherapy can also be administered postoperatively: 1) when the drug is instilled from the first to the 4th-5th postoperative days, with infusions every 24 hours without hyperthermia, is called Early Postoperative Intraperitoneal Chemotherapy (EPIC); 2) if the intraperitoneal chemotherapy is administered by cycles, weeks or months following CRS, is called Normothermic IntraPEritoneal Chemotherapy (NIPEC). Without being a chemotherapy treatment, an Extensive Intraoperative Peritoneal Lavage (EIPL) is considered another intraperitoneal treatment. Besides, intraperitoneal chemotherapy can be combined with systemic chemotherapy as neoadjuvant therapy before surgery to attempt to decrease the extent of PM; this bidirectional method with neoadjuvant intraperitoneal and systemic chemotherapy is called NIPS. Finally, Pressurized IntraPeritoneal Aerosol Chemotherapy (PIPAC) is a closed technique of chemotherapy administration; it is a new technique that has been used in palliative scenarios for symptoms control or as neoadjuvant therapy, with promising results.

The type of drug to be used will depend on the way of intraperitoneal delivery. For HIPEC, LHIPEC or PIPAC, the cancer chemotherapeutic agents must have rapid cytotoxic effects and must not be cell-cycle specific, because they are administered for a short time (1 or 2 hours or less) [3]; for HIPEC or LHIPEC, the drug must also have synergism with heat. However, the chemotherapy drugs for EPIC, NIPEC or NIPS may be cell-cycle specific because they are instilled for long time periods [3].

HIPEC

HIPEC consists of the intraoperative intraperitoneal administration of chemotherapy, usually after CRS. The local administration of chemotherapy allows the instillation of high doses of drugs without increasing systemic complications. The agents used in HIPEC must have high molecular weight to prevent their penetration through the PPB into the bloodstream [2]; the anticancer drug must also have synergism with heat because it is instilled in the carrier solution when a temperature of 41-43°C is reached. Hyperthermia has a cytotoxic effect by itself, especially in the high mitotic index tumor cells [4, 5]. Additionally, heat increases drug penetration capacity into the tissues [2, 3, 5–9].

HIPEC is administered in a single intraoperative cycle, ensuring compliance with treatment in almost 100% of patients. Cytotoxicity of the drugs used in HIPEC must be independent of the cell cycle in order to act on all malignant cells regardless of the phase of the cell cycle in which they are. The most common drugs used in PM from GC origin are Cisplatin (with or without Doxorubicin) and Mitomycin-C, alone or in combination; the dose for Cisplatin varies between 50 to 200 mg/m2 during 60 to 90 minutes, and for Mitomycin-C the dose most commonly used is 30–40 mg during 60–120 minutes [1, 10–14]. Oxaliplatin is also used with a dose of 460 mg/m2 during 30 minutes [11, 15, 16].

HIPEC can be administered by different techniques, being the best known the open and closed techniques [1]. In the open technique (Sugarbaker coliseum), a retractor is used to elevate the patient abdominal wall and the HIPEC circulation system is placed with the skin open (Figure 1); this system allows a direct visualization of the abdomen during the instillation facilitating its manipulation to distribute the drug to all parietal and visceral peritoneal surfaces, but it has a greater heat loss and a greater risk of spillage and exposition to the operation room staff [2]. In the closed technique, the catheters are placed with the skin edges temporarily closed by a continuous suture; the desired temperature is achieved more quickly due to a lesser heat dispersion, and the spillage risk is minimized, but it has the problem of the non-uniform abdominal distribution of the drug [3]. The distribution can be improved by the introduction of CO2 gas bubbles that produce a turbulent flow of the perfusion (Figure 2), achieving an homogeneous distribution within the abdomen [3, 17]. The use of one or other method of administration does not seem to influence the survival results or the morbidity associated with the procedure, as has been shown in a recent study from United States comparing both techniques in 1812 patients [18].

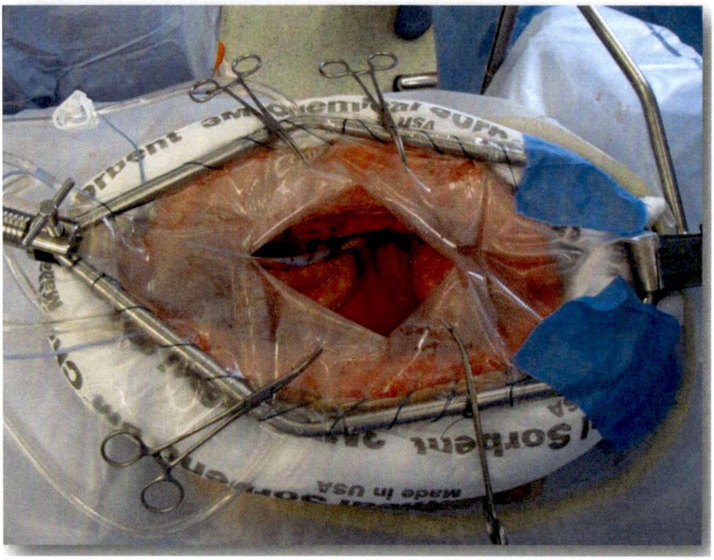

Figure 1. Open technique (Sugarbaker coliseum) for HIPEC administration.

Focused on GC, HIPEC can be administered for the treatment of established PM from GC or as prophylactic treatment in patients with locally advanced GC to prevent peritoneal recurrence. As has been said, laparoscopic HIPEC (LHIPEC) can also be used as neoadjuvant therapy or as palliative treatment.

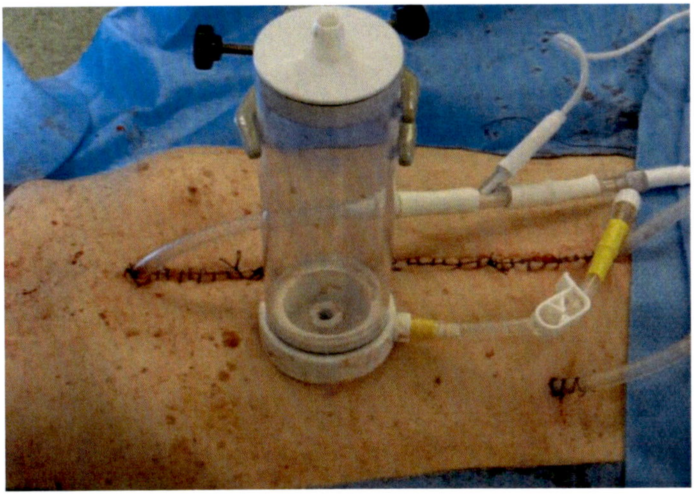

Figure 2. Closed technique with CO2 recirculation for HIPEC administration.

HIPEC for Treatment of established PM from GC

The combination of SCT with CRS (including curative gastrectomy, D2 lymphadenectomy and resection of all peritoneal implants) and HIPEC is the treatment with the best published results for patients with PM from GC [19]. The main studies are summarized in Table 1.

The most common HIPEC drugs for PM from GC are Cisplatin (with or without Doxorubicin) and Mitomycin-C, alone or in combination, with the doses already mentioned [1, 10, 19]. Oxaliplatin is also used with the dose noted above [1, 11, 15, 19].

There are several retrospective series and case-control studies that show a potential benefit with CRS and HIPEC. Even, there is one randomized clinical trial published in 2011 by Yang et al. They randomized 68 patients to be treated with CRS alone or with CRS associated with HIPEC (with a combination of Mitomycin-C and Cisplatin). They reported a significant but modest improvement in survival when HIPEC was associated to CRS, with a median OS of 11 months versus 6.5 months for CRS without HIPEC, with 3-year OS of 5.9% and 0% respectively [12].

There are three published National Registries with a high volume of patients in western countries. The French Registry was published in 2010 by Glehen et al. [15] with 159 patients from 15 centers; they reported a median OS of 9.2 months (1-, 3- and 5-year survival of 43%, 18% and 13%, respectively). When the CRS was complete, with no tumoral residue, the median OS reached 15 months. The authors recommended that patients with a Peritoneal Cancer Index (PCI) [20] higher than 12 should not been treated with CRS and HIPEC, as survival in these patients was the same as with SCT.

The Spanish Registry was published in 2019 [11]. This registry included 88 patients from 7 specialized Spanish Institutions. With a median follow-up of 32 months, the median OS was 21.2 months. The median OS at 1-year was 79.9% and at 3-year 30.9%. The patients with PCI 0–6 had the best results with a median OS of 26.1 months (1-, 3- and 5-year survival of 88.7%, 46.8% and 46.8%, respectively), compared to 18.9 months of median OS in patients with PCI > 6 (1-, 3- and 5-year survival of 70.4%, 15.1% and 0%, respectively). These differences were significant in the comparative analysis with a HR of 2.23 (95% CI: 1.28–3.88, $p = 0.003$).

The German Registry was published recently, in 2020 [21]. This study included 235 patients from 38 centers. The authors described a median OS of 13 months, but the OS rose to 18 months in the group of patients with PCI 0–6. The best results have been reached in high volume centers (with more than 20 patients included in the study); the OS in experienced centers is significantly better than in low volume centers (16 versus 12 months, $p = 0.02$).

In 2019, Bonnot et al. published the French propensity score study CYTO-CHIP [22], comparing 180 patients treated with CRS and HIPEC versus 97 patients treated only with CRS. The patients treated with HIPEC had better survival than those treated without HIPEC, with a median OS of 18.8 versus 12.1 months, without morbidity and mortality differences.

Currently, there are several Asian trials recruiting patients. The German phase III trial GASTRIPEC (NCT02158988) was closed on July 4, 2018 due to low recruitment, according to the presentation made at the

PSOGI International Congress in Paris in September 2018, but there is one ongoing Dutch clinical trial (PERISCOPE II, NCT03348150) evaluating the role of HIPEC for PM of GC. In a few years, we will have more information from these trials that are currently underway [19].

Table 1. Published studies evaluating hyperthermic intraperitoneal chemotherapy (HIPEC) as treatment of peritoneal metastases from gastric cancer [19]

Author. Year	Number of patients	Drug	Morbidity	Survival
Yonemura. 1996 [6]	83 (CRS + HIPEC)	MMC + Cisplatin + Etoposide	NA	5-year OS: 11%
Fujimoto. 1997 [23]	48 (CRS + HIPEC) vs. 18 (CRS)	MMC	NA	5-year OS: 31% vs. 0%, p = 0.001
Glehen. 2010 [15]	159 (CRS + HIPEC)	MMC, Cisplatin, Oxaliplatin	Grade 3-4: 27.8%. Mortality: 6.5%	Median OS: 9.2 months. 5-year OS: 13%
Yang. 2011 [12]	34 (CRS + HIPEC) vs. 34 (CRS)	MMC + Cisplatin	14.7% vs. 11.7%. Mortality: 0%	Median OS: 11 vs. 6.5 months
Manzanedo. 2019 [11]	88 (CRS + HIPEC)	Cisplatin, Doxorubicin, MMC, Oxaliplatin	Severe morbidity: 31%. Mortality: 3.4%	Median OS: 21.2 months. 3-year OS: 30.9%
Bonnot. 2019 [22]	180 (CRS + HIPEC) vs. 97 (CRS)	MMC, Cisplatin, Oxaliplatin	53.7% vs. 55.3%. Mortality: 7.4% vs. 10.1%	Median OS: 18.8 vs. 12.1 months. 5-year OS: 19.9% vs. 6.4%
Rau. 2020 [21]	235 (CRS + HIPEC)	MMC, Cisplatin, Doxorubicin, Oxaliplatin	Severe morbidity: 17%. Mortality: 5.1%	Median OS: 13 months. 5-year OS: 6%

CRS: Cytoreductive surgery; HIPEC: Hyperthermic Intraperitoneal Chemotherapy; MMC: Mitomycin C; NA: Not available; OS: Overall survival.

HIPEC as Neoadjuvant Treatment

Intraperitoneal chemotherapy can be used in GC with PM as neoadjuvant treatment to reduce the peritoneal disease burden in order to increase the number of patients in whom complete cytoreduction can be achieved [19].

The preoperative use of LHIPEC has been recently studied [24, 25]. In 2017, Yonemura et al. reported 53 patients treated with 2 neoadjuvant cycles of LHIPEC (with a combination of Docetaxel plus Cisplatin). The benefit of the treatment was evaluated according to the results of peritoneal cytology and PCI determination. A significant PCI reduction was observed (from a median PCI of 14.2 to 11.8 in the second session) and the cytology changed from positive to negative in 68% of patients. Moreover, 8 patients (15%) showed a complete disappearance of the peritoneal disease [24].

In 2019, Badgwell et al. published a phase-II trial with 19 patients. They used LHIPEC with a combination of Mitomycin-C 30 mg and Cisplatin 200 mg (1–5 preoperative cycles). The peritoneal disease (macroscopic and microscopic disease) disappeared in 7 patients after the last LHIPEC cycle with a very low rate of morbidity (11%) after 38 total procedures. They reported a median OS of 20.3 months and OS at 3 years of 43.5% [25].

LHIPEC can be used as neoadjuvant treatment in GC with PM because its results are promising with acceptable morbidity [1].

HIPEC as Prophylactic or Adjuvant Treatment

The peritoneal relapse is the most common pattern of recurrence of locally advanced GC after radical treatment with surgery (gastrectomy plus D2 lymphadenectomy) and intensive perioperative SCT. The association of HIPEC to a curative gastrectomy, in patients with a locally advanced GC without PM, can prevent peritoneal relapse. Several Asian studies have demonstrated that the use of HIPEC as a prophylactic treatment is safe and effective [19]. The main published studies evaluating the role of HIPEC as a prophylactic treatment are summarized in Table 2.

Table 2. Published studies evaluating hyperthermic intraperitoneal chemotherapy (HIPEC) as prophylactic treatment in high risk patients without peritoneal metastases [19]

Author. Year	Number of patients	Drug	Morbidity	Survival
Koga. 1988 (26)	26 (surgery + HIPEC) vs. 21 (surgery alone)	MMC	Anastomotic leak: 3.1% vs. 7.1%	30-month OS: 83% vs. 67%
Ikeguchi. 1995 (30)	78 (surgery + HIPEC) vs. 96 (surgery alone)	MMC	1.2% vs. 2.1%	5-year OS: 51% vs. 46%
Fujimoto. 1999 (31)	71 (surgery + HIPEC) vs. 70 (surgery alone)	MMC	2/71 vs. 2/70	4-year OS: 76% vs. 58%
Yonemura. 2001 (16)	48 (surgery + HIPEC) vs. 44 (surgery + NIPEC) vs. 47 (surgery alone)	MMC + Cisplatin	19% vs. 14% vs. 19% (mortality: 4% vs. 0% vs. 4%)	5-year OS: 61% vs. 44% vs. 42%
Zhu. 2006 (32)	41 (surgery + HIPEC) vs. 53 (surgery alone)	MMC+ Cisplatin	23% vs. 12%	4-year OS: 70% vs. 52%
Coccolini. Meta-analysis 2014 (28)	116 (surgery + HIPEC) vs. 88 (surgery alone)	MMC, Cisplatin	Morbidity rate better in surgery group (OR = 1.82)	2-year OS: Better in HIPEC (OR = 0.24)
Desiderio. Meta-analysis 2017 (13)	731 (surgery + HIPEC) vs. 1079 (surgery alone)	MMC, cisplatin, etoposide	Higher risk in HIPEC group (RR = 2.17)	5-year OS better in HIPEC (RR = 0.82)

Koga et al. published for the first time the long-term benefit of HIPEC as adjuvant treatment. They reported their results in 1988, with a significant improvement in survival (3-years OS of 74% in HIPEC group versus 53% in non-HIPEC group) [26].

In 2001, Yonemura et al. randomized 139 patients in three groups (surgery alone, surgery plus NIPEC and surgery with HIPEC) and the survival results at 5-year were 61% in the HIPEC group versus 44% and 42% in the two other groups ($p = 0.02$) [16].

The survival benefit of adjuvant HIPEC has been confirmed in different reviews and meta-analyses [13, 19, 27, 28]. In 2007, Yan et al. performed a review of 13 studies and their results showed a survival benefit when HIPEC was added to surgery (HR = 0.60; $p = 0.002$) [27]. Recently, in 2017, Desiderio et al. published a meta-analysis of 11 clinical trials and 21 observational studies, with more than 2,500 patients. The 5-year OS for patients treated with adjuvant HIPEC was better than that of the patients treated with surgery alone (RR = 0.82, $p = 0.01$) [13].

For prophylactic use of HIPEC, most of the published studies are Asian, and perhaps this is the reason why its use has not been extended to Western countries. Nevertheless, currently a new important clinical trial is ongoing in Europe (GASTRICHIP) and we will know if its outcomes are similar to the Asian studies when the results become available [29].

HIPEC as Palliative Treatment

Many patients with PM from GC have unresectable disease, and these cases can develop malignant ascites which can result in numerous symptoms such as abdominal pain, dyspnea, early satiety, or fatigue.

LHIPEC is an option for these patients. Some studies have reported a success rate in symptom control of 95% [33, 34]. Valle et al. in 2009 published the results of 52 patients (15 of them with GC) with refractory malignant ascites treated with palliative LHIPEC. They reported a complete disappearance of the ascites in 94% of patients without severe morbidity [33].

In 2012, Facchiano et al. published a systematic review which included 76 patients treated with palliative LHIPEC. They reported a 95% success in ascites control, with 7% mild complications and without severe morbidity [34].

LHIPEC is a safe treatment with a high rate of success in ascites control and can be considered a real option for these patients.

EPIC

The administration of intraperitoneal chemotherapy in the immediate postoperative period is called EPIC; the drug is instilled from the first to the 4th-5th postoperative days, with infusions every 24 hours without hyperthermia; EPIC is administered and recovered through an inflow catheter and drains placed during the CRS [19]. The EPIC regimens include cell-cycle specific drugs, such as Melphalan, Taxanes or 5-Fluorouracil [1, 19], because EPIC is administered in repeated applications for a longer time that allows the drug to be in contact with tumor cells in their different cell phases (unlike HIPEC).

Yu et al. published the results of a prospective randomized trial in 2001. They randomized 248 patients with GC without PM to receive standard surgery with or without EPIC (with Mitomycin-C plus 5-Fluorouracil) as adjuvant treatment. The EPIC group had better 5-year OS (54% versus 38%, $p = 0.028$) [35].

In 2014, Kwon et al. published the results of a retrospective study with 245 patients diagnosed by locally advanced (serosal invasion) GC without PM; 180 patients were treated with surgery alone and 65 patients with surgery plus EPIC. The addition of EPIC decreased peritoneal relapses (18.5% in EPIC group versus 32.2% in non-EPIC group, $p = 0.04$) and thus OS was better (5-year OS of 47.4% in EPIC group and 26.7% in non-EPIC group, $p = 0.01$) [36].

EPIC can be added to CRS and HIPEC in patients with good performance status in experienced centers [10, 19]. However, the use of EPIC is not as widespread as that of HIPEC, because it can generate more infections, fistulas, or other postoperative complications [19].

NIPEC

NIPEC consists in the administration of intraperitoneal chemotherapy weeks or months after CRS, by several cycles at body temperature. A catheter to administrate the drug is placed into the abdominal cavity, usually after CRS. The chemotherapeutic agent used for NIPEC may be a cell-cycle specific drug with a high molecular weight that allows it to remain for long periods of time in the peritoneal cavity. Paclitaxel is the drug most commonly administrated. Gemcitabine, pemetrexed or 5-fluorouracil are safe and effective drugs for NIPEC too. Doxorubicin, Mitomycin-C or Melphalan are not recommended for NIPEC [3].

There are few studies on this type of intraperitoneal chemotherapy administration, which are limited to case series, and even fewer in GC. As noted above, in 2001 Yonemura et al. compared three prophylactic treatments to prevent peritoneal relapses in advanced GC without PM; they randomized 139 patients in three groups (surgery alone, surgery plus NIPEC and surgery with HIPEC) and the 5-year OS was 61% in HIPEC group versus 44% and 42% in the two other groups ($p = 0.02$) [16]; therefore, NIPEC did not show benefits over surgery alone in OS.

In addition, NIPEC has the problem that is poorly distributed in the presence of intestinal adhesions, which are very frequent after extensive abdominal surgery. For all these reasons, more studies are needed to demonstrate its efficacy as it has been shown in ovarian cancer.

Extensive Intraoperative Peritoneal Lavage (EIPL)

EIPL consists of washing the abdominal cavity after CRS with a large amount of saline solution (first with 1 liter that is completely aspirated, repeating this washing 10 more times). This type of intraperitoneal treatment was reported by Kuramoto et al. for patients with GC and positive peritoneal cytology [1]. The aim of this lavage is to eliminate the cancer cells that may remain floating in the peritoneal cavity [37].

Kuramoto et al. published in 2009 a randomized controlled trial of 88 patients with GC. The patients were randomized to surgery alone, surgery plus NIPEC and surgery plus NIPEC and EIPL. The study showed a significant increase in OS in the EIPL group, with a median OS of 35 months versus 15 and 16 months in the other groups [38].

However, a recent Chinese randomized clinical trial [39] did not observe the hypothetical value of EIPL in this setting.

NIPS

In 2006, Yonemura et al. reported the multimodal combination of neoadjuvant intraperitoneal and systemic chemotherapy (NIPS) in patients with GC and PM [40]. A peritoneal port system is placed into the abdominal cavity, and a combination of intraperitoneal Taxotere plus Carboplatin with intravenous Methotrexate and 5-Fluorouracil is administered (between 2 and 6 cycles).

The results published by Yonemura in 2006 showed that NIPS achieved a negative peritoneal cytology in 56% of patients and 38 of 61 patients showed a partial response [40].

Later, in 2012, Yonemura et al. published the results of NIPS with intraperitoneal Taxotere and Cisplatin combined with systemic S-1. Ninety-six patients were enrolled in the study and 82 patients were eligible for CRS. Complete cytoreduction (CCS-0) was achieved in 70% and 36.8% of patients had complete pathologic response [41].

Other studies have shown similar results with different NIPS regimens. Fujiwara et al. published the results of NIPS in 25 patients; 56% of patients had a complete regression of PM with a significant OS increase in the patients with complete response of peritoneal disease (27.1 months versus 9.6 months) [42].

NIPS can be a neoadjuvant option of treatment for selected patients in experimented centers.

PIPAC

PIPAC is a new technique devised to improve the quality of life for patients with unresectable PM [19]. Pressurized intraperitoneal aerosol chemotherapy (PIPAC) is a closed technique of chemotherapy administration. The chemotherapy is administered by laparoscopy, aerosolized by an injector at high pressure, so that it achieves a better penetration into the tissues [43].

In the last years, many studies have been published about PIPAC. All the studies are focused on palliative patients. In 2019, Alyami et al. published a systematic review of 838 patients (185 of them with GC). The symptoms control rate was 50 to 91% in patients with GC [44]. Currently, there are many ongoing studies evaluating the use of PIPAC for PM, even considering its use as a neoadjuvant treatment to test the possibility of achieving a complete cytoreduction in initially unresectable patients. There are great expectations about PIPAC, both in the palliative setting and as neoadjuvant therapy. The results published so far are encouraging, but they are no better than those of LHIPEC, which is a safe and widely studied treatment (neoadjuvant as well as palliative), and it is frankly cheaper [19]. Therefore, future studies should compare PIPAC with LHIPEC to really know if PIPAC provides better outcomes than those already demonstrated by LHIPEC.

References

[1] Macrì A, Morabito F. The use of intraperitoneal chemotherapy for gastric malignancies. *Expert Rev Anticancer Ther.* 2019;19(10):879-88.

[2] González-Moreno S, González-Bayón LA, Ortega-Pérez G. Hyperthermic intraperitoneal chemotherapy: Rationale and technique. *World J Gastrointest Oncol.* 2010;2(2):68-75.

[3] Sugarbaker PH. Intraperitoneal delivery of chemotherapeutic agents for the treatment of peritoneal metastases: current challenges and

how to overcome them. *Expert Opin Drug Deliv.* 2019;16(12):1393-401.

[4] Sticca RP, Dach BW. Rationale for hyperthermia with intraoperative intraperitoneal chemotherapy agents. *Surg Oncol Clin N Am.* 2003;12(3):689-701.

[5] Elias DM, Ouellet JF. Intraperitoneal chemohyperthermia: rationale, technique, indications, and results. *Surg Oncol Clin N Am.* 2001;10(4):915-33, xi.

[6] Yonemura Y, Fujimura T, Nishimura G, FallaR null, Sawa T, Katayama K, et al. Effects of intraoperative chemohyperthermia in patients with gastric cancer with peritoneal dissemination. *Surgery.* 1996;119(4):437-44.

[7] Sugarbaker PH. Peritoneal Metastases from Gastrointestinal Cancer. *Curr Oncol Rep.* 2018;20(8):62.

[8] Sugarbaker PH. Laboratory and clinical basis for hyperthermia as a component of intracavitary chemotherapy. *Int J Hyperthermia.* 2007;23(5):431-42.

[9] Jacquet P, Averbach A, Stuart OA, Chang D, Sugarbaker PH. Hyperthermic intraperitoneal doxorubicin: pharmacokinetics, metabolism, and tissue distribution in a rat model. *Cancer Chemother Pharmacol.* 1998;41(2):147-54.

[10] Gamboa AC, Winer JH. Cytoreductive Surgery and Hyperthermic Intraperitoneal Chemotherapy for Gastric Cancer. *Cancers.* 2019;11(11).

[11] Manzanedo I, Pereira F, Rihuete Caro C, Pérez-Viejo E, Serrano Á, Gutiérrez Calvo A, et al. Cytoreductive Surgery and Hyperthermic Intraperitoneal Chemotherapy (HIPEC) for Gastric Cancer with Peritoneal Carcinomatosis: Multicenter Study of Spanish Group of Peritoneal Oncologic Surgery (GECOP). *Ann Surg Oncol.* 2019;26(8):2615-21.

[12] Yang X-J, Huang C-Q, Suo T, Mei L-J, Yang G-L, Cheng F-L, et al. Cytoreductive surgery and hyperthermic intraperitoneal chemotherapy improves survival of patients with peritoneal

carcinomatosis from gastric cancer: final results of a phase III randomized clinical trial. *Ann Surg Oncol.* 2011;18(6):1575-81.

[13] Desiderio J, Chao J, Melstrom L, Warner S, Tozzi F, Fong Y, et al. The 30-year experience-A meta-analysis of randomised and high-quality non-randomised studies of hyperthermic intraperitoneal chemotherapy in the treatment of gastric cancer. *Eur J Cancer.* 2017;79:1-14.

[14] Yonemura Y, Kawamura T, Bandou E, Takahashi S, Sawa T, Matsuki N. Treatment of peritoneal dissemination from gastric cancer by peritonectomy and chemohyperthermic peritoneal perfusion. *Br J Surg.* 2005;92(3):370-5.

[15] Glehen O, Gilly FN, Arvieux C, Cotte E, Boutitie F, Mansvelt B, et al. Peritoneal carcinomatosis from gastric cancer: a multi-institutional study of 159 patients treated by cytoreductive surgery combined with perioperative intraperitoneal chemotherapy. *Ann Surg Oncol.* 2010;17(9):2370-7.

[16] Yonemura Y, de Aretxabala X, Fujimura T, Fushida S, Katayama K, Bandou E, et al. Intraoperative chemohyperthermic peritoneal perfusion as an adjuvant to gastric cancer: final results of a randomized controlled study. *Hepatogastroenterology.* 2001;48 (42):1776-82.

[17] Sánchez-García S, Villarejo-Campos P, Padilla-Valverde D, Amo-Salas M, Martín-Fernández J. Intraperitoneal chemotherapy hyperthermia (HIPEC) for peritoneal carcinomatosis of ovarian cancer origin by fluid and CO2 recirculation using the closed abdomen technique (PRS-1.0 Combat): A clinical pilot study. *Int J Hyperthermia.* 2016;32(5):488-95.

[18] Leiting JL, Cloyd JM, Ahmed A, Fournier K, Lee AJ, Dessureault S, et al. Comparison of open and closed hyperthermic intraperitoneal chemotherapy: Results from the United States hyperthermic intraperitoneal chemotherapy collaborative. *World J Gastrointest Oncol.* 2020;12(7):756-67.

[19] Manzanedo I, Pereira F, Serrano Á, Pérez-Viejo E. Review of management and treatment of peritoneal metastases from gastric cancer. *J Gastrointest Oncol.* 2020. doi:10.21037/jgo-20-232.

[20] Portilla AG, Shigeki K, Dario B, Marcello D. The intraoperative staging systems in the management of peritoneal surface malignancy. *J Surg Oncol.* 2008;98(4):228-31.

[21] Rau B, Brandl A, Piso P, Pelz J, Busch P, Demtröder C, et al. Peritoneal metastasis in gastric cancer: results from the German database. *Gastric Cancer.* 2020;23(1):11-22.

[22] Bonnot P-E, Piessen G, Kepenekian V, Decullier E, Pocard M, Meunier B, et al. Cytoreductive Surgery With or Without Hyperthermic Intraperitoneal Chemotherapy for Gastric Cancer With Peritoneal Metastases (CYTO-CHIP study): A Propensity Score Analysis. *J Clin Oncol.* 2019;37(23):2028-40.

[23] Fujimoto S, Takahashi M, Mutou T, Kobayashi K, Toyosawa T, Isawa E, et al. Improved mortality rate of gastric carcinoma patients with peritoneal carcinomatosis treated with intraperitoneal hyperthermic chemoperfusion combined with surgery. *Cancer.* 1997;79(5):884-91.

[24] Yonemura Y, Ishibashi H, Hirano M, Mizumoto A, Takeshita K, Noguchi K, et al. Effects of Neoadjuvant Laparoscopic Hyperthermic Intraperitoneal Chemotherapy and Neoadjuvant Intraperitoneal/Systemic Chemotherapy on Peritoneal Metastases from Gastric Cancer. *Ann Surg Oncol.* 2017;24(2):478-85.

[25] Badgwell B, Blum M, Das P, Estrella J, Wang X, Ho L, et al. Phase II Trial of Laparoscopic Hyperthermic Intraperitoneal Chemoperfusion for Peritoneal Carcinomatosis or Positive Peritoneal Cytology in Patients with Gastric Adenocarcinoma. *Ann Surg Oncol.* 2017;24(11):3338-44.

[26] Koga S, Hamazoe R, Maeta M, Shimizu N, Murakami A, Wakatsuki T. Prophylactic therapy for peritoneal recurrence of gastric cancer by continuous hyperthermic peritoneal perfusion with mitomycin C. *Cancer.* 1988;61(2):232-7.

[27] Yan TD, Black D, Sugarbaker PH, Zhu J, Yonemura Y, Petrou G, et al. A systematic review and meta-analysis of the randomized controlled trials on adjuvant intraperitoneal chemotherapy for resectable gastric cancer. *Ann Surg Oncol.* 2007;14(10):2702-13.

[28] Coccolini F, Cotte E, Glehen O, Lotti M, Poiasina E, Catena F, et al. Intraperitoneal chemotherapy in advanced gastric cancer. Meta-analysis of randomized trials. *Eur J Surg Oncol.* 2014;40(1):12-26.

[29] Glehen O, Passot G, Villeneuve L, Vaudoyer D, Bin-Dorel S, Boschetti G, et al. GASTRICHIP: D2 resection and hyperthermic intraperitoneal chemotherapy in locally advanced gastric carcinoma: a randomized and multicenter phase III study. *BMC Cancer.* 2014;14:183.

[30] Ikeguchi M, Kondou A, Oka A, Tsujitani S, Maeta M, Kaibara N. Effects of continuous hyperthermic peritoneal perfusion on prognosis of gastric cancer with serosal invasion. *Eur J Surg.* 1995;161(8):581-6.

[31] Fujimoto S, Takahashi M, Mutou T, Kobayashi K, Toyosawa T. Successful intraperitoneal hyperthermic chemoperfusion for the prevention of postoperative peritoneal recurrence in patients with advanced gastric carcinoma. *Cancer.* 1999;85(3):529-34.

[32] Zhu ZG, Tang R, Yan M, Chen J, Yang QM, Li C, et al. Efficacy and safety of intraoperative peritoneal hyperthermic chemotherapy for advanced gastric cancer patients with serosal invasion. A long-term follow-up study. *Dig Surg.* 2006;23(1-2):93-102.

[33] Valle M, Van der Speeten K, Garofalo A. Laparoscopic hyperthermic intraperitoneal peroperative chemotherapy (HIPEC) in the management of refractory malignant ascites: A multi-institutional retrospective analysis in 52 patients. *J Surg Oncol.* 2009;100(4):331-4.

[34] Facchiano E, Risio D, Kianmanesh R, Msika S. Laparoscopic hyperthermic intraperitoneal chemotherapy: indications, aims, and results: a systematic review of the literature. *Ann Surg Oncol.* 2012;19(9):2946-50.

[35] Yu W, Whang I, Chung HY, Averbach A, Sugarbaker PH. Indications for early postoperative intraperitoneal chemotherapy of advanced gastric cancer: results of a prospective randomized trial. *World J Surg.* 2001;25(8):985-90.

[36] Kwon OK, Chung HY, Yu W. Early postoperative intraperitoneal chemotherapy for macroscopically serosa-invading gastric cancer patients. *Cancer Res Treat.* 2014;46(3):270-9.

[37] Yonemura Y, Canbay E, Li Y, Coccolini F, Glehen O, Sugarbaker PH, et al. A comprehensive treatment for peritoneal metastases from gastric cancer with curative intent. *Eur J Surg Oncol.* 2016; 42(8):1123-31.

[38] Kuramoto M, Shimada S, Ikeshima S, Matsuo A, Yagi Y, Matsuda M, et al. Extensive intraoperative peritoneal lavage as a standard prophylactic strategy for peritoneal recurrence in patients with gastric carcinoma. *Ann Surg.* 2009;250(2):242-6.

[39] Misawa K, Mochizuki Y, Sakai M, Teramoto H, Morimoto D, Nakayama H, et al. Randomized clinical trial of extensive intraoperative peritoneal lavage versus standard treatment for resectable advanced gastric cancer (CCOG 1102 trial). *Br J Surg.* 2019;106(12):1602-10.

[40] Yonemura Y, Bandou E, Sawa T, Yoshimitsu Y, Endou Y, Sasaki T, et al. Neoadjuvant treatment of gastric cancer with peritoneal dissemination. *Eur J Surg Oncol.* 2006;32(6):661-5.

[41] Yonemura Y, Elnemr A, Endou Y, Ishibashi H, Mizumoto A, Miura M, et al. Effects of neoadjuvant intraperitoneal/systemic chemotherapy (bidirectional chemotherapy) for the treatment of patients with peritoneal metastasis from gastric cancer. *Int J Surg Oncol.* 2012;2012:148420.

[42] Fujiwara Y, Takiguchi S, Nakajima K, Miyata H, Yamasaki M, Kurokawa Y, et al. Neoadjuvant intraperitoneal and systemic chemotherapy for gastric cancer patients with peritoneal dissemination. *Ann Surg Oncol.* 2011;18(13):3726-31.

[43] Esquis P, Consolo D, Magnin G, Pointaire P, Moretto P, Ynsa MD, et al. High intra-abdominal pressure enhances the penetration and antitumor effect of intraperitoneal cisplatin on experimental peritoneal carcinomatosis. *Ann Surg.* 2006;244(1):106-12.

[44] Alyami M, Hübner M, Grass F, Bakrin N, Villeneuve L, Laplace N, et al. Pressurised intraperitoneal aerosol chemotherapy: rationale, evidence, and potential indications. *Lancet Oncol.* 2019;20(7):e368-77.

In: Gastric Peritoneal Carcinomatosis
Editors: F. López Mozos et al.
ISBN: 978-1-53619-487-6

Chapter 9

Current Role of PIPAC in Peritoneal Metastases of Gastric Origin

M. C. Fernández*, MD, M. E. Barrios, MD and F. López, PhD
Upper Gastrointestinal and Peritoneal Oncology Surgery Unit
Department of Surgery
Hospital Clínico Universitario – Valencia (Spain)

Abstract

Pressurized intraperitoneal aerosol chemotherapy (PIPAC) is a novel method of intraperitoneal drug-delivery with the capability of distributing drugs as a pressurized aerosol. The first clinical use of this method was described by M.A. Reymond in Germany in November, 2011 [1]. In this chapter we summarize the characteristics of this technique, its indications and the current evidence published in the treatment of patients with peritoneal metastases from gastric cancer.

* Corresponding Author's E-mail: mcfm89@gmail.com.

Rationale of PIPAC

Peritoneal metastases (PM) involve a poor prognosis with a reduced response to systemic chemotherapy compared with other metastatic sites [2]. In this setting, cytoreductive surgery with hyperthermic intraperitoneal chemotherapy (HIPEC) improves long-term outcomes in selected patients [3]. However, low tissue penetration and no homogeneous distribution are the main limiting factors for the efficacy of intraperitoneal chemotherapy with fluids [4].

These pharmacokinetic problems in peritoneal drug administration are not considered in PIPAC therapy due to its different pharmacological properties. Aerosols are a suspension of liquid droplets in a gas and gases distribution is homogeneous within a closed space [5]. Then, the drug tissue concentration will be higher than the reported after HIPEC (Table 1). Furthermore, the aerosol is applied to the abdominal cavity under pressure so an artificial pressure gradient is created between the intraperitoneal space and the interstitium of the peritoneal tumour [6]. Then, the drug tissue penetration will be improved (Table 1).

Table 1. Main advantages of PIPAC drug-administration method

Solass et al. [1]	Tissue Concentration	Tissue Penetration
Doxorubicin (liquid)	0.02 μmol/g	10-30 μm
Doxorubicin (aerosol)	0.03–4.1 μmol/g	500-700 μm

Surgical Technique for PIPAC

PIPAC is performed by laparoscopic approach under general anesthesia and in a supine position. A normothermic capnoperitoneum with a pressure between 12 and 15 mmHg is generated. Then, a 5-mm and 12-mm balloon trocars are inserted.

First, a staging laparoscopy determining the peritoneal cancer index (PCI) is performed. Biopsies from all 4 quadrants are taken to histological examination and a local peritonectomy is sometimes carried out to improve accuracy of anatomopathology. Ascities can be suctioned off and peritoneal cytology may be taken.

To disperse the chemotherapy as pressurized aerosol, a nebulizer is connected to an intravenous high–pressure injector and inserted into the abdomen through a trocar.

It is essential to avoid any exposure of the operating time taking overall three safety measures. First, the system has to be checked for tightness. Second, the operating room should be equipped with laminar air flow. Third, the chemotherapy application is a remote-controlled process and nobody remain in the operating room during the application.

When the operating room is not equipped with laminar air flow, a transparent plastic cover protection connected to a smoke filtration device has been used as an alternative (Figure 1). The safety of this technique has been described by Delhorme et al. [7].

It is mandatory an operational security check-list protocol and it must be double-checked before PIPAC administration. Chemotherapeutic solution is aerosolized during 30 minutes, the system must be stay closed and with a pressure between 13 and 20 bar (= 200 to 300 psi). Then, the aerosol is suctioned off through a closed exhaust system and disposed of.

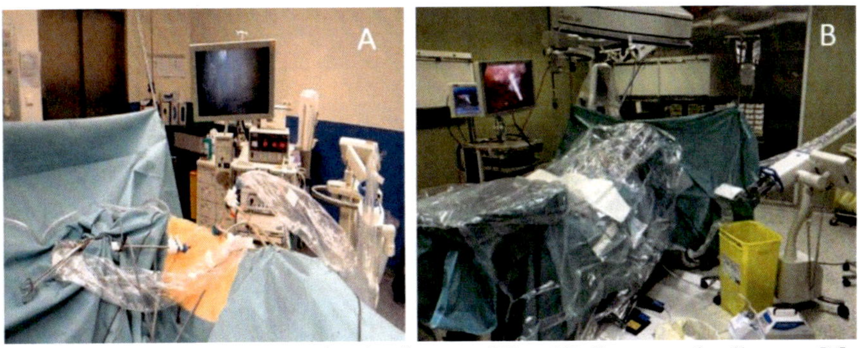

Pictures reprinted from Reymond and colleagues [8] and Delhorme and colleagues [7].

Figure 1. PIPAC with (A) and without (B) laminar air flow in the operating room.

INDICATIONS

Current indications of PIPAC consist on the palliative treatment of isolated PM as second- or third-line treatment if there is tumour progression under systemic chemotherapy [9–12]. In a recent systematic review, 1,810 PIPAC procedures in 838 patients were included. 41% of the indications for PIPAC were for PM of ovarian cancer, 22% for gastric cancer, 12% for colorectal cancer, 7% for peritoneal mesothelioma and 17% for other indications, in particular hepatobiliary and pancreatic tumors [13].

Other indications for PIPAC are intolerance or severe side effects of palliative systemic chemotherapy, patient's refusal of systemic chemotherapy, or organ toxicity (e.g., kidney failure) that precludes the further use of platinum-based chemotherapeutic agents (Table 2).

Table 2. Summary of current indications for PIPAC therapy

≥ 3rd line in ovarian cancer
≥ 2nd line in gastric cancer
≥ 2nd line in hepatobiliary cancer
Recurrence malignant peritoneal mesothelioma
Salvage situation in colorectal cancer
Ascites control in the platin-resistant patients
Intolerance/ side-effects of systemic chemotherapy

Recently, it has been proposed the role of PIPAC as neoadjuvant therapy. Alyami et al. suggest that PIPAC therapy can lead to CRS and HIPEC. They performed secondary CRS and HIPEC in 14.4% of 406 patients with unresectable PM after neoadjuvant PIPAC treatments. 66.7% of these patients were alive and with no recurrence in a median follow-up of 7 months [14]. Girshally et al. showed that in nine patients with unresectable PM, an objective radiological and histological tumor regression were observed after repeated PIPAC (mean number of cycles 3.5 ± 0.9) and leading to CRS and HIPEC [15].

It is essential to rule out the conditions in which PIPAC must be avoided. Absolute contraindications for PIPAC therapy are: short life expectancy, bowel obstruction, total parenteral nutrition or gastric drainage, decompensated ascites and simultaneous intestinal anastomosis and PIPAC. Other extraperitoneal metastases, ECOG > 2, portal vein thrombosis, previous CRS and HIPEC and previous anaphylactic reaction to the drug used are relative contraindications that must be considered.

Treatment Regimen and Assessment of Response

Two intraperitoneal regimens are used for PIPAC procedures: cisplatin in combination with doxorubicin (10.5 mg/m2 and 2.1 mg/m2, respectively) and oxaliplatin as monotherapy (92 mg/m2). At least three PIPAC procedures are usually repeated at 6 ± 2-week intervals. The interval can possibly be increased to 12 weeks if there is high-grade or complete histological regression. Treatment discontinuation must be considered in presence of peritoneal tumor progression, development of visceral metastases and/or toxicity.

Combination of PIPAC with systemic chemotherapy is possible with most used regimens, including FOLFOX, FOLFIRI, FLOT, and EOX. It is recommended pause systemic treatment for 2 weeks before and 1 week after PIPAC procedure [16]. In case of the systemic administration of angiogenesis inhibitors, a 4-week pause is recommended because of the known risk of sometimes lethal bowel perforations [17].

PIPAC has been performed as a hospital treatment with a median hospital stay of three days [12, 18], but a recent study shows the safety of PIPAC as an outpatient procedure [19].

Treatment response can be assessed macroscopically, radiologically and histologically.

- Macroscopic criteria: determination of “Peritoneal Cancer Index” (PCI) before every PIPAC sessions.

- Radiological criteria: Repeated CT scans are performed at 3 to 6 months interval, and radiological response is assessed according to RECIST criteria [20].
- Histological criteria: histological comparison of sequential biopsies before the individual applications of PIPAC using the "Peritoneal Regression Grading System (PRGS)" is the most suitable method to assess tumor regression [21]. The PRGS includes the following 4 categories: Grade 1: complete response (absence of tumor cells), Grade 2: major response (major regression features, few residual tumor cells), Grade 3: minor response (some regressive features but predominance of residual tumor cells), Grade 4: no response (tumor cells without any regression features).

ROLE OF PIPAC IN PERITONEAL METASTASES OF GASTRIC CANCER. CURRENT EVIDENCE

One of the first controlled studies on efficacy and safety of PIPAC with cisplatin and doxorubicin (PIPAC C/D) included the patients with recurrent gastric cancer with peritoneal metastases and disease progression after at least one line of previous intravenous chemotherapy. This trial evaluated tumor response with histology and laparoscopy (PCI), it showed a high rate of objective histological regression. Mean PCI remained stable under PIPAC C/D therapy but they insist on the difficulties to distinguish visually between vital PM and avital scarring. PIPAC therapy was also well tolerated with no mortality and no severe adverse events [22].

In combination with systemic chemotherapy (XELOX, FLOT), PIPAC has also been studied as first-line treatment for PM of gastric cancer. PIPAC with intraperitoneal cisplatin and doxorubicin combined with palliative systemic chemotherapy with XELOX has demonstrated that it is active in patients with PM from gastric cancer and with histological tumor response in 60 % of patients [23]. Furthermore, therapy with PIPAC showed a low rate of complications, there were no serious adverse events and no mortality. The same work group presented its results in a retrospective case series of 24 patients with PM from gastric cancer treated by PIPAC alone with lower histological regression rates (50%) than with systemic chemotherapy [24].

Gockel et al. [25] included the patients with PM from gastric cancer excluded for CRS and HIPEC taking into account the PCI (usually higher than 8–10), comorbidities, and patients' preferences. Patients with progressive disease during systemic chemotherapy were not eligible for PIPAC in this study. They showed PIPAC as a palliative therapy able to alleviate symptoms, in particular to control ascites and to induce (partial) macroscopic and histological regression of PM, leading to a better quality of life.

Including patients with chemotherapy-resistant PM from gastric cancer, Ellebæk et al. demonstrated that PIPAC with low-dose cisplatin and doxorubicin can induce objective tumour response and with encouraging survival data [26]. In this study, the objective histological response and stable disease was documented in 40% and 20%, respectively, after two PIPAC directed treatments. The median overall survival after the diagnosis was 11.5 months while this was 4.7 months after the first PIPAC procedure. These results are similar to the experiences from German centres [22] with an overall survival of 6.7 months and a complete or major regression on histology in 36% of patients.

Finally, Alyami et al. presented a median survival of 19.1 months [27]. These results for patients with gastric peritoneal metastasis are promising when compared with data for patients who have been treated with systematic chemotherapy alone, in whom the reported median survival did not exceed 10.7 months (95% CI 9·1–12·8) [28]. This retrospective serie also presents a mortality of 4.7%, one related to small bowel obstruction and the other from a pulmonary embolism. Another point to mention is that six patients became resectable after a median of 3 PIPAC and underwent curative intent CRS and HIPEC.

Table 3. Summary of current publications for PIPAC in peritoneal metastases of gastric cancer

Study/Year	Therapy	n	PIPAC procedures	Histological response	Toxicity
Phase-II studies					
Khomyakov et al., 2016 [23]	PIPAC C/D + XELOX	31	56	Complete response (PRGS1) 4/15 (27%) Partial response (PRGS2) 5/15 (33%) No response (PRGS 3 and 4) 6/15 (40%)	Diaphragmatic perforation (n = 1) Nausea (n = 3) Mortality 0%
Struller et al., 2019 [22]	PIPAC C/D	25	43	Complete response (PRGS1) 1/12 (8.3%) Partial response (PRGS2) 8/12 (66.7%) No response (PRGS 3 and 4) 3/12 (25%)	Subileus (n = 2) Abdominal pain (n = 25) Hypoalbuminemia (n = 1) Vomiting (n = 1) Liver toxicity (n = 1) Subcutaneous toxic emphysema (n = 1) Mortality 0%
Retrospective series					
Nadiradze et al., 2016 [24]	PIPAC C/D	24	60	Complete response 6/17 (35.3%) Partial response 6/17 (35.3%) No response 5/17 (29.4%)	Ascities descompensation (n = 1) Nausea and emesis (n = 1) Allergy reaction (n = 1) Hepatotoxicity (n = 7) Abdominal pain (n = 6) Mortality 0%

Study/Year	Therapy	n	PIPAC procedures	Histological response	Toxicity
Gockel et al., 2018 [25]	PIPAC C/D	24	46	Decreased % of tumor cells 7/14 (50%) Stable % of tumor cells 4/14 (28.6%) Increased % of tumor cells 3/14 (21.4%)	Nausea and emesis (n = 1) Mortality 0%
Ellebæk et al., 2020 [26]	PIPAC C/D +/- systemic chemotherapy	20	52	Complete response (PRGS1) 0/10 (0%) Partial response 5/10 (50%) No response or stable 5/10 (50%)	Minor reversible neuropathy Urinary retention Nausea and emesis Wound dehiscence (n = 1) Mortality 0%
Alyami et al., 2020 [27]	PIPAC C/D + systemic chemotherapy	42	163	N/A	Ascities drainage (n = 1) Intestinal obstruction (n = 1) Allergy reaction (n = 2) Pulmonary embolism (n = 1) Abdominal pain (n = 5) Mortality 4.7%

Future Perspectives

PIPAC appears to be safe and well tolerated. However, it remains difficult to assess the effectiveness of this method without randomized trials at this time.

The first randomized trials of patients with PM from ovarian or gastrointestinal cancers are already being conducted (NCT04329494) and the primary outcome is to assess the dose limiting toxicities.

Some of the phase II studies currently ongoing including patients with PM from gastric cancer are:

- PIPAC in combination with standard chemothcrapy in primarily untreated naive upper GI-adenocarcinomas with peritoneal seeding (phase II/III trial) and the primary outcome is to evaluate its oncologic efficacy (EudraCT: 2018-001035-40) [29].
- Treatment of peritoneal carcinomatosis with Pressurized IntraPeritoneal Aerosol Chemotherapy - PIPAC-OPC2. It includes patients with PM from gastrointestinal, ovarian or primary peritoneal cancer. The primary outcome of this study is to evaluate if PIPAC can induce major or complete response (PRGS 1 or 2) within a series of three PIPAC procedures [30].
- A randomized and multicentre phase II study of PIPAC with cisplatin and doxorubicin in gastric PM (PIPAC EstoK 01), the primary endpoint is progression-free survival [31].

Some of the current questions with regard to PIPAC therapy are being investigated. But for now, PIPAC should only be performed within the framework of clinical studies when competing with an evidence-based therapy.

REFERENCES

[1] Solass W, Kerb R, Mürdter T, Giger-Pabst U, Strumberg D, Tempfer C, Zieren J, Schwab M, Reymond M A. Intraperitoneal chemotherapy of peritoneal carcinomatosis using pressurized aerosol as an alternative to liquid solution: first evidence for efficacy. *Ann. Surg. Oncol.* 2014;21:553–559.

[2] Franko J, Shi Q, Meyers J P, et al. Prognosis of patients with peritoneal metastatic colorectal cancer given systemic therapy: an analysis of individual patient data from prospective randomised trials from the Analysis and Research in Cancers of the Digestive System (ARCAD) database. *Lancet Oncol.* 2016; 17: 1709–19.

[3] Glehen O, Gilly F N, Boutitie F, et al. Toward curative treatment of peritoneal carcinomatosis from nonovarian origin by cytoreductive surgery combined with perioperative intraperitoneal chemotherapy: a multi-institutional study of 1290 patients. *Cancer* 2010; 116: 5608–18.

[4] Dedrick R L, Flessner M F. Pharmacokinetic problems in peritoneal drug administration: tissue penetration and surface exposure. *J. Natl. Cancer Inst* 1997; 89: 480–87.

[5] Fick A. Über diffusion. *Ann. Phys.* 1855;94:59–86.

[6] Esquis P, Consolo D, Magnin G, Pointaire P, Moretto P, Ynsa M D, Beltramo J L, Drogoul C, Simonet M, Benoit L, Rat P, Chauffert B. High intraabdominal pressure enhances the penetration and antitumor effect of intraperitoneal cisplatin on experimental peritoneal carcinomatosis. *Ann. Surg.* 2006;244:106–12.

[7] Delhorme J B, Klipfel A, D'Antonio F, Greget M C, Diemunsch P, Rohr S, Brigand C. Occupational safety of pressurized intraperitoneal aerosol chemotherapy (PIPAC) in an operating room without laminar airflow. *J. Visc. Surg.* 2019. doi:10.1016/j.jviscsurg.2019.06.010.

[8] N/A.

[9] Tempfer C B, Rezniczek G A, Ende P, Solass W, Reymond M A. Pressurized Intraperitoneal Aerosol Chemotherapy with cisplatin and

doxorubicin in women with peritoneal carcinomatosis: a cohort study. *Anticancer Res.* 2015;35:6723–9.

[10] Demtröder C, Solass W, Zieren J, Strumberg D, Giger-Pabst U, Reymond M A. Pressurized intraperitoneal aerosol chemotherapy with oxaliplatin in colorectal peritoneal metastasis. *Color Dis.* 2016;18:364–71.

[11] Graversen M, Detlefsen S, Bjerregaard J K, Pfeiffer P, Mortensen M B. Peritoneal metastasis from pancreatic cancer treated with pressurized intraperitoneal aerosol chemotherapy (PIPAC). *Clin. Exp. Metastasis.* 2017;34:309–14.

[12] Nowacki M, Alyami M, Villeneuve L, Mercier F, Hubner M, Willaert W, et al. Multicenter comprehensive methodological and technical analysis of 832 pressurized intraperitoneal aerosol chemotherapy (PIPAC) interventions performed in 349 patients for peritoneal carcinomatosis treatment: an international survey study. *Eur. J. Surg. Oncol.* 2018;44:991–6.

[13] Alyami M, Hübner M, Grass F, Bakrin N, Villeneuve L, Laplace N, Passot G, Glehen O, Kepenekian V. Pressurised intraperitoneal aerosol chemotherapy: rationale, evidence, and potential indications. Lancet Oncol. 2019 Jul;20(7):e368-e377. doi: 10.1016/S1470-2045(19) 30318-3.

[14] Alyami M, Mercier F, Siebert M, Bonnot P E, Laplace N, Villeneuve L, Passot G, Glehen O, Bakrin N, Kepenekian V. Unresectable peritoneal metastasis treated by pressurized intraperitoneal aerosol chemotherapy (PIPAC) leading to cytoreductive surgery and hyperthermic intraperitoneal chemotherapy. *Eur. J. Surg. Oncol.* 2019 Jun 21:S0748-7983(19)30522-0. doi: 10.1016/j.ejso. 2019.06.028.

[15] Girshally R, Demtröder C, Albayrak N, Zieren J, Tempfer C, Reymond MA. Pressurized intraperitoneal aerosol chemotherapy (PIPAC) as a neoadjuvant therapy before cytoreductive surgery and hyperthermic intraperitoneal chemotherapy. *World J. Surg. Oncol.* 2016 Sep 27;14(1):253. doi: 10.1186/s12957-016-1008-0.

[16] Robella M, Vaira M, De Simone M. Safety and feasibility of pressurized intraperitoneal aerosol chemotherapy (PIPAC) associated with systemic chemotherapy: an innovative approach to treat peritoneal carcinomatosis. *World J. Surg. Oncol.* 2016;14:128.

[17] Qi W X, Shen Z, Tang L N, Yao Y. Bevacizumab increases the risk of gastrointestinal perforation in cancer patients: a meta-analysis with a focus on different subgroups. *Eur. J. Clin. Pharmacol.* 2014;70:893–906.

[18] Alyami M, Gagniere J, Sgarbura O, Cabelguenne D, Villeneuve L, Pezet D, Quenet F, Glehen O, Bakrin N, Passot G. Multicentric initial experience with the use of the pressurized intraperitoneal aerosol chemotherapy (PIPAC) in the management of unresectable peritoneal carcinomatosis. *Eur. J. Surg. Oncol.* 2017 Nov;43(11):2178-2183. doi: 10.1016/j.ejso.2017.09.010.

[19] Graversen M, Lundell L, Fristrup C, Pfeiffer P, Mortensen M B. Pressurized IntraPeritoneal Aerosol Chemotherapy (PIPAC) as an outpatient procedure. *Pleura Peritoneum.* 2018;3(4):20180128. doi:10.1515/pp-2018-0128.

[20] Eisenhauer E A, Therasse P, Bogaerts J, et al. New response evaluation criteria in solid tumours: revised RECIST guideline (version 1.1). *Eur. J. Cancer* 2009; 45: 228–47.

[21] Solass W, Sempoux C, Carr N Y, Detlefsen S, Bibau F. Peritoneal sampling procedures and histological assessment of therapeutic response: proposal of the Peritoneal Regression Grading Score (PRGS). *Pleura Peritoneum.* 2016;1:99–107.

[22] Struller F, Horvath P, Solass W, Weinreich F J, Strumberg D, Kokkalis M K, Fischer I, Meisner C, Königsrainer A, Reymond M A. Pressurized intraperitoneal aerosol chemotherapy with low-dose cisplatin and doxorubicin (PIPAC C/D) in patients with gastric cancer and peritoneal metastasis: a phase II study. *Ther. Adv. Med. Oncol.* 2019 May 13;11:1758835919846402. doi: 10.1177/1758835919 846402.

[23] Khomyakov V, Ryabov A, Ivanov A, Bolotina L, Utkina A, Volchenko N, Kaprin A. Bidirectional chemotherapy in gastric

cancer with peritoneal metastasis combining intravenous XELOX with intraperitoneal chemotherapy with low-dose cisplatin and Doxorubicin administered as a pressurized aerosol: an open-label, Phase-2 study (PIPAC-GA2). *Pleura Peritoneum.* 2016 Sep 1;1(3):159-166. doi: 10.1515/pp-2016-0017.

[24] Nadiradze G, Giger-Pabst U, Zieren J, Strumberg D, Solass W, Reymond M A. Pressurized Intraperitoneal Aerosol Chemotherapy (PIPAC) with low-dose cisplatin and doxorubicin in gastric peritoneal metastasis. *J. Gastrointest. Surg.* 2016;20:367–73.

[25] Gockel I, Jansen-Winkeln B, Haase L, Rhode P, Mehdorn M, Niebisch S, Moulla Y, Lyros O, Lordick F, Schierle K, Wittekind C, Thieme R. Pressurized Intraperitoneal Aerosol Chemotherapy (PIPAC) in Gastric Cancer Patients with Peritoneal Metastasis (PM): Results of a Single-Center Experience and Register Study. *J. Gastric. Cancer.* 2018 Dec;18(4):379-391. doi: 10.5230/jgc.2018.18.e37.

[26] Ellebæk S B, Graversen M, Detlefsen S, Lundell L, Fristrup C W, Pfeiffer P, Mortensen M B. Pressurized intraperitoneal aerosol chemotherapy (PIPAC) of peritoneal metastasis from gastric cancer: a descriptive cohort study. *Clin. Exp. Metastasis.* 2020 Apr;37(2):325-332. doi: 10.1007/s10585-020-10023-5.

[27] Alyami M, Bonnot P E, Mercier F, Laplace N, Villeneuve L, Passot G, Bakrinab N, Kepenekianab V, Glehen O. Pressurized intraperitoneal aerosol chemotherapy (PIPAC) for unresectable peritoneal metastasis from gastric cancer. *Eur. J. Surg. Oncol.* 2020.

[28] Al-Batran S E, Homann N, Pauligk C, Illerhaus G, Martens U M, Stoehlmacher J, et al. Effect of Neoadjuvant Chemotherapy Followed by Surgical Resection on Survival in Patients With Limited Metastatic Gastric or Gastroesophageal Junction Cancer: The AIO-FLOT3 Trial. *JAMA Oncol.* 2017;3(9):1237-44.

[29] Oliver Goetze T, Al-Batran S E, Pabst U, Reymond M, Tempfer C, Bechstein W O, Bankstahl U, Gockel I, Königsrainer A, Kraus T, Mönig S P, Rau B, Schwarzbach M, Piso P. Pressurized intraperitoneal aerosol chemotherapy (PIPAC) in combination with standard of care chemotherapy in primarily untreated chemo naïve

upper gi-adenocarcinomas with peritoneal seeding - a phase II/III trial of the AIO/CAOGI/ACO. *Pleura Peritoneum.* 2018 Jun 8;3(2):20180113. doi: 10.1515/pp-2018-0113.

[30] Graversen M, Detlefsen S, Asmussen J, et al. Treatment of peritoneal carcinomatosis with Pressurized IntraPeritoneal Aerosol Chemotherapy - PIPAC-OPC2. *Pleura Peritoneum.* 2018;3(2): 20180108. doi:10.1515/pp-2018-0108.

[31] Eveno C, Jouvin I, Pocard M. PIPAC EstoK 01: Pressurized IntraPeritoneal Aerosol Chemotherapy with cisplatin and doxorubicin (PIPAC C/D) in gastric peritoneal metastasis: a randomized and multicenter phase II study. *Pleura Peritoneum.* 2018 Jun 21;3(2):20180116. doi: 10.1515/pp-2018-0116.

In: Gastric Peritoneal Carcinomatosis
Editors: F. López Mozos et al.
ISBN: 978-1-53619-487-6

Chapter 10

Scientific Advances and Future Perspectives

Areeba Saif, MD and Andrew Blakely*, MD
Center for Cancer Research, National Cancer Institute,
NIH, Bethesda, Washington, US

Abstract

Over the last decade, despite advances in the management of peritoneal carcinomatosis, there remains a lack of a standardized treatment approach that confers a meaningful survival benefit in those with gastric cancer. However, there are several innovative diagnostic and therapeutic modalities on the horizon. In this chapter, we discuss novel serum and peritoneal biomarkers of peritoneal metastasis, advances in traditional diagnostic imaging and fluorescence guided intraoperative detection of peritoneal metastasis. Total neoadjuvant therapy is discussed as an attractive solution for patients who are rendered unsuitable for any additional adjuvant treatment following surgical resection in part secondary to the significant post-operative morbidity experienced by them. A shift in the approach to gastric cancer treatment from a generalized 'trial and error' method to a more personalized targeted

* Corresponding Author's E-mail: andrew.blakely@nih.gov.

treatment strategy is highlighted by discussing aspects of existing cell/tissue models, genetically engineered murine models, patient derived xenografts/patient-derived orthotopic xenograft, patient derived gastric cancer organoids and the SMART System (Sample Microenvironment from Resected Metastatic Tumors) - A Human, Immunocompetent Tumor Platform. Regarding immunotherapy, a brief overview of immune check-point blockade such as PD-1/PD-L1, CTLA-4, Tim-3 or IDO is provided. Adoptive Cell Therapy, Combinational Immunotherapy, Cancer Vaccines, Nanoparticle Drug Delivery System, Photodynamic therapy and Cell-free and concentrated ascites reinfusion therapy (CART) are also described and discussed.

INTRODUCTION

Despite significant advances in the treatment of peritoneal disease secondary to intra-abdominal malignancies, peritoneal metastasis (PM) in gastric cancer (GC) continues to confer a dismal prognosis with a median survival approaching 2.8 to 3.1 months [1]. Up to 45% of patients with gastric adenocarcinoma will develop PM during the course of their disease [2], and while cytoreductive surgery (CRS) and hyperthermic intraperitoneal chemotherapy (HIPEC) have shown benefit in a highly selected population of GC patients, the optimal management of peritoneal disease from GC remains controversial. In this chapter, we will review the emerging landscape of diagnostic and therapeutic modalities in managing GC with PM.

EMERGING SCREENING AND DIAGNOSTIC TOOLS IN GASTRIC CANCER WITH PERITONEAL METASTASIS

Novel Peritoneal and Serum Biomarkers

Peritoneal metastasis are often difficult to diagnose using standard imaging modalities. While the established gold standard for diagnosis of PM is a diagnostic laparoscopy, it lacks the sensitivity to detect microscopic involvement. Peritoneal lavage with cytologic examination is the traditional method to detect free tumor cells, but it also has limited sensitivity and is reported to miss more than half of cytology-positive cases [3]. Hence, there has been increasing focus on identifying novel diagnostic approaches that complement peritoneal lavage cytology. Reverse-transcriptase polymerase chain reaction (RT-PCR) detection of biomarkers in peritoneal lavage has been used to increase the sensitivity of diagnosis of PM. Chen et al., published a review of existing biomarkers that not only increase the sensitivity of PM detection but may also have prognostic significance, including: CEA [4, 5], CA12-5 [6], CK20 [7], Ber-EP4 [8-10], MMP-7 [11, 12], survivin [5], MUC2 [5], IL-17 [13)], FABP1, TFF1, and MASPIN [14,15]. While CEA is the most frequently reported marker, identifying these biomarkers through molecular diagnostics to detect PM in peritoneal lavage fluid has mostly been assessed in retrospective cohort studies. There has also been recent interest in the examination of GC-derived peritoneal exosomes in peritoneal fluid, with Ohzawa et al., reporting the association of reduced expression of exosomal miR-29s with synchronous and metachronous PM in GC with serosal involvement [16].

Several studies have also explored the possibility of using blood-borne markers with high sensitivity and specificity that may reliably indicate the presence of PM and as such have made a case for the so-called 'liquid biopsy.' In a study published in the *Annals of Surgical Oncology*, circulating tumor DNA (ctDNA) was found to be a promising marker for treatment selection, prognostication, and surveillance after definitive therapy in patients with PM. Patients with high levels of perioperative ctDNA and new postoperative ctDNA alterations had worse outcomes following resection of PM [17]. MicroRNAs (miRs), which are short, non-coding RNAs responsible for regulating mRNAs, have also been studied as potential biomarkers. A study reported plasma exosome-encapsulated microRNA-21 and microRNA-92a as promising biomarkers for the prediction of peritoneal recurrence in patients with GC [18].

Additional research is needed to identify and validate both peritoneal and serum biomarkers, especially through prospective trials, to establish their clinical feasibility and validity in detecting peritoneal disease. This will hopefully make PM and its recurrence less challenging to diagnose in the future.

Gastric Peritoneal Metastasis Predictive Models and Advances in Traditional Diagnostic Modalities

Cytoreductive surgery (CRS) and hyperthermic intraperitoneal chemotherapy (HIPEC) have shown mixed results in patients with PM in gastric cancer, with only those patients who have a low peritoneal disease burden and can undergo a complete cytoreduction (CC) experiencing the greatest survival benefit. Hence, the identification of patients who will benefit most from CRS and HIPEC is essential in the management of gastric cancer patients with PM.

While traditional imaging modalities may have low sensitivity for the detection of PM, several predictive models have been developed to increase their diagnostic sensitivity. Kim et al., developed a CT-based predictive model using multivariate logistic regression that evaluated tumor size, presence of Borrmann type 4 disease or *linitis plastica*, lymphadenopathy, indirect findings of PM (peritoneal thickening, fat stranding, plaques or nodules on the peritoneum, and ascites), and definitive findings of PM (omental caking and rectal shelf) [19]. The objective of this model was to use CT imaging to risk-stratify patients with GC for risk of PM and to thereby better select who should undergo staging laparoscopy versus definitive surgical treatment. They found that tumor size >5.2 cm, Borrmann type 4, enlarged lymph node(s), peritoneal plaques or nodules, and ascites were independently associated with PM and this model was able to predict PM with a higher sensitivity than definitive findings of PM on CT (sensitivity 92.3% vs. 38.3%). Therefore, patients without definitive imaging findings of PM but with other concerning features were recommended to undergo staging laparoscopy, while those without concerning features were recommended to undergo definitive resection.

Radiomic analysis using contrast-enhanced CT to preoperatively predict PM in patients with advanced gastric cancer has been reported. Radiomics is a method that uses data-characterization algorithms to extract a large number of features from radiographic images. This approach has the potential to identify distinctive imaging features that may be missed by the naked eye. A venous-phase CT radiomics model was developed by Liu et al., which used six venous-phase features on CT to predict GC with peritoneal metastasis. [20]. While CT-based T stage was found to be an independent predictor of PM in advanced gastric cancer, the radiomics model showed worse diagnostic efficacy than the clinicopathological model used by the authors, which incorporated information such as primary tumor location in the stomach, grade, and histology. However, predictive models based on CT driven radiomics do hold promise in improving the diagnostic accuracy of conventional noninvasive imaging modalities.

Researchers have also used artificial intelligence to develop a CT-based deep learning model to predict PM in patients with gastric cancer. This ongoing clinical trial will use a deep convolutional neural network (DCNN) model to retrospectively analyze CT scans from patients who were initially diagnosed as PM-negative on CT but were found to have peritoneal disease on surgery or laparoscopy. This study aims to significantly increase the sensitivity of CT in diagnosing PM [21].

Intraoperatively, the peritoneal cancer index (PCI) is the most widely used score for patient-stratification in determining which patients will undergo CRS and HIPEC; however, it is often limited by inter-observer variability. A Gastric Cancer Peritoneal Carcinomatosis Risk Score has been created by researchers at the Loma Linda University using patient-level data from the California Cancer Registry [1]. The score determines the risk of PM based on the cumulative effect of high-risk features including age, sex, race/ethnicity, clinical T stage, grade, anatomic subsite, and presence or absence of signet-ring histology. The score has several limitations including the omission of nodal status, which is a strong predictor of peritoneal disease. It remains to be seen whether this score will have wide-spread adoption and clinical relevance following prospective validation of the score.

Fluorescence-Guided Intraoperative Detection of Peritoneal Metastasis

There has been ongoing research to identify biomarker targets for intraoperative fluorescence imaging of peritoneal implants to aid surgical resection. Epithelial cell adhesion molecule (EpCAM) and carcinoembryonic antigen (CEA) have been identified as suitable targets for fluorescence imaging of PM in patients with colorectal cancer. In a study conducted by Hoogstins et al., overexpression of EpCAM and CEA was seen in 100% of PM samples and the expression was strong in >70% of samples in patients from colorectal cancer [22]. No similar targets have been identified in clinical studies at present for peritoneal metastasis from gastric cancer but the identification of markers that reliably indicate PM would significantly improve the detection of PM in patients with gastric cancer.

Indocyanine green (ICG) is an agent capable of emitting fluorescence and preferentially accumulates in tumor tissue. ICG-based fluorescence imaging has been used to identify the draining lymph nodes in early gastric cancer [23, 24]. Subsequent work has evaluated ICG-based intraoperative imaging for detecting peritoneal nodules. A systematic review of seven series using ICG-based detection of peritoneal metastasis reported sensitivity ranging from 72.4 to 100% and specificity from 54.2 to 100% [25].

Considerations for Re-Staging after Intraperitoneal Therapy

As increasing numbers of GC patients are evaluated for and undergo intraperitoneal therapy for either synchronous or metachronous PM, another key aspect of interval or post-treatment clinical re-staging will be to reliably differentiate treated non-tumor-bearing scar versus persistent, viable tumor nodules or plaques. While generous or numerous biopsies may provide some information regarding persistent peritoneal disease, improved targeting of such biopsies will minimize sampling error and over-or under-assessment of patients' true disease burdens. This in turn allows for optimal triaging of said patients to either additional intraperitoneal therapy, surgical treatment, or investigational therapies. This may represent an opportunity for machine learning to assist in real-time differentiation of scar versus tumor, building on growing experiences in using machine learning for assessing the ability to completely cytoreduce patients at the time of diagnostic laparoscopy [26].

Multimodality Therapy for Metastatic Gastric Cancer – Prospects and Recent Advances

The emergence of precision medicine and an improved understanding of the heterogeneous landscape of gastric cancer has led to significant efforts not only to optimize the current chemotherapeutic regimens but also to develop targeted molecular therapy in an effort to expand treatment options and provide a meaningful survival benefit to patients with metastatic gastric cancer. This section will provide an overview of recent advances in the multimodal management of gastric cancer with PM.

Total Neoadjuvant Therapy

While perioperative chemotherapy and surgery are now standard of care for locally advanced gastric cancer as established by the MAGIC trial, there remains a substantial risk of non-administration, dose reduction, or incomplete adjuvant therapy for many patients, in part secondary to significant postoperative morbidity following surgical resection for gastric cancer [27]. Total neoadjuvant chemotherapy (TNT) presents an attractive solution to this problem. However, there has been concern about the tolerability of prolonged neoadjuvant chemotherapy (NAC) or chemoradiotherapy (NACRT) regimens and their subsequent impact on perioperative morbidity and mortality in patients who go on to receive surgical treatment.

The NeoFLOT study is a phase II multicenter study that investigated the application of prolonged neoadjuvant chemotherapy in patients with locally advanced gastroesophageal cancer (GEC) [28)]. Each of the 59 enrolled patients in the study received 6 cycles of 5-fluorouracil, leucovorin, oxaliplatin, and docetaxel (FLOT) every 2 weeks prior to undergoing surgery. R0 resection, which was the primary endpoint of the study, was 86%. Ganchow et al., went on to analyze the impact of intensified NACT on perioperative outcomes in patients undergoing surgery for GEC [29]. Out of the 537 patients enrolled in the study, 132 patients received chemotherapy under the standard neoadjuvant protocol, 356 patients received no chemotherapy, and 49 patients underwent intensified chemotherapy as per the NeoFLOT trial. They reported no significant increase in perioperative complications in patients receiving intensified NACT with 6 preoperative cycles of FLOT.

Several studies have reported similarly promising results for TNT. Roeland et al., in a retrospective study, demonstrated TNT followed by resection is feasible and has an acceptable 57.1% rate of TNT completion [30]. In a study [31] conducted at The Memorial Sloan Kettering Cancer Center, USA, Greally et al., compared postoperative length of stay (LOS) and surgical morbidity between patients who received perioperative chemotherapy versus patients who received TNT [31]. They reported no significant differences in LOS or surgical morbidity in the two groups. Moreover, patients in the TNT group received higher proportions of the planned treatment compared to patients in the perioperative treatment group, demonstrating a potential benefit of administering chemotherapy in a neoadjuvant setting.

Although there is retrospective data demonstrating the efficacy and safety of TNT, there is a lack of published prospective trial data to further support this approach. An ongoing phase II clinical trial (NCT04062058) of TNT for locally advanced gastric cancer may bridge this gap. This study is designed to evaluate the rate of pathologic complete response of neoadjuvant chemoradiotherapy and neoadjuvant chemotherapy followed by surgery for locally advanced gastric adenocarcinoma. While most of these studies exclude patients with peritoneal metastasis, TNT is a promising avenue and will perhaps in the future have a wider application for more advanced stages of gastric cancer, possibly using a bidirectional treatment approach.

Immunotherapy

Given recent advances in molecular biology, there has been a shift in the approach to gastric cancer treatment from a generalized 'trial and error' method to a more personalized targeted treatment strategy. Immunotherapy, both as monotherapy and in combination with antitumoral targeted agents, has emerged as a promising option for personalized management of advanced gastric cancer. Immune checkpoint inhibitors (ICI), adoptive cell transfer (ACT), chimeric antigen receptor T cells (CAR-T cells), immunotoxin treatment, and vaccine-based therapies have all been investigated as potential treatment strategies for gastric cancer and peritoneal metastasis.

Immune Checkpoint Blockade

Immune checkpoint (IC) blockade, especially programmed cell death-1 (PD-1) and its ligand (PD-L1), has shown efficacy in the management of advanced gastric cancer, including chemo-refractory gastric cancer. Based on the results of the phase II KEYNOTE-059 clinical trial, pembrolizumab (an anti-PD-1 monoclonal antibody) was approved by the Food and Drug Administration (FDA) of the United States of America (USA) for treatment of advanced gastric adenocarcinoma expressing PDL1 [33]. Other ICI including the anti-PD-1 nivolumab, the anti-PD-L1 agent avelumab, and the CTLA-4 inhibitors ipilimumab and tremelimumab have also been studied in locally advanced unresectable upper gastrointestinal cancers [34]. Additionally, several IC proteins are currently being investigated as potential therapeutic targets in preclinical and clinical studies including lymphocyte-activation gene 3 protein (LAG-3), T-cell immunoglobulin domain and mucin domain (TIM-3), and T-cell immunoreceptor with immunoglobulin and ITIM domains (TIGIT) [35, 36], Wang et al., performed multiplex profiling of peritoneal metastasis from GC in 43 patients to identify novel targets and molecular subtypes predictive of treatment response and reported that the less treatment responsive 'mesenchymal-like' subtype of PM was associated with high expression of TIM-3, galectin-9, VISTA, and TGF-β1, which could be potential targets for IC blockade [2].

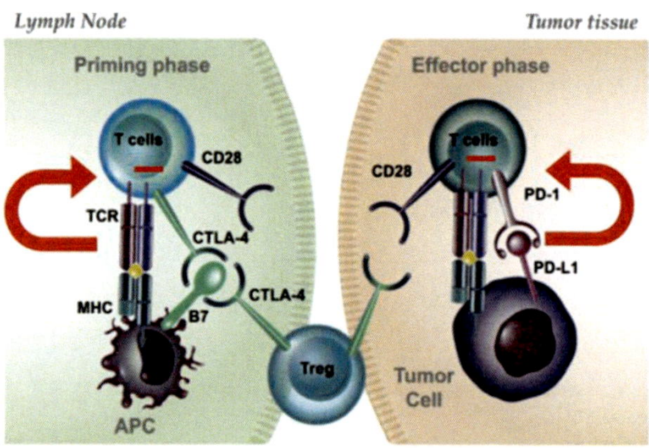

	CTLA-4	PD-1
Receptor distribution	Secondary lymphoid organs	Inflamed/injured peripheral tissues, secondary lymphoid organs
Target T cells	Recently primed T cells	Effector T cells
Phosphatases	SHP-1, SHP-2, PP2a	SHP-2
Metabolic changes	Glycolysis inhibition	Glycolysis inhibition, FAO induction

Figure 1. Differences between CTLA-4 and PD-1 Immune Inhibitory Pathway. Schematic representation of CTLA-4 and PD-1 molecular functions. Different outcomes of these molecular pathways in tumor-bearing hosts may be mechanistically explained at least at four levels: expression pattern and localization, expression kinetic during T cell activation, partner phosphatases in the downstream signaling pathway, and metabolic effects. TCR, T cell receptor; MHC, major histocompatibility class molecules; FAO, fatty acid oxidation; Treg, regulatory T cell. Figure reproduced with permission from Zappasodi et al., [32].

Intraperitoneal immunotherapy has also been considered an attractive option for the management of not only peritoneal metastasis but also malignant ascites arising secondary to PM. Catumaxomab is a bispecific and trifunctional antibody with two different antigen-binding sites, EpCAM, CD3, and a functional Fc domain that binds to and activates types I, IIa, and III Fcγ-receptors on NK cells [37]. It has been approved by the FDA for the treatment of refractory malignant ascites in patients with PM. In a pilot study including 8 patients with malignant ascites due to peritoneal disease, intraperitoneal administration of Catumaxomab resulted in complete elimination of tumor cells and the disappearance of ascites in all patients [38]. In a prospective randomized phase II/III trial, Heiss et al., randomized 258 patients with malignant ascites due to epithelial cancer into two arms: paracentesis plus catumaxomab or paracentesis alone. In the catumaxomab group, median puncture-free survival was significantly longer in addition to improved overall survival in patients with gastric cancer [39]. The most common adverse event was cytokine-release syndrome secondary to increased levels of increase of IL-6 and TNF-alpha [37)]. At present, Catumaxomab is the only bispecific antibody approved for clinical application.

Adoptive T-Cell Therapy

Chimeric antigen receptor (CAR) T-cell therapy is another promising immunotherapeutic avenue currently under investigation for gastric cancer and peritoneal metastasis. CAR-T immunotherapy uses genetically engineered T cells that have an extracellular single-chain variable fragment (scFv) against specific cancer antigens of interest and a T-cell activating domain [40]. T cells are obtained from a patient's blood, then genetically modified to introduce the chimeric antigen receptor (CAR), giving them the ability to recognize specific tumor-associated antigens, and then infused back in the patient. Some of the identified targets for CAR-T cell immunotherapy in gastric cancer include HER2, CEA, MUC1, EpCAM, CLDN 18.2, MSLN, NKG2D, and FOLR1 [41].

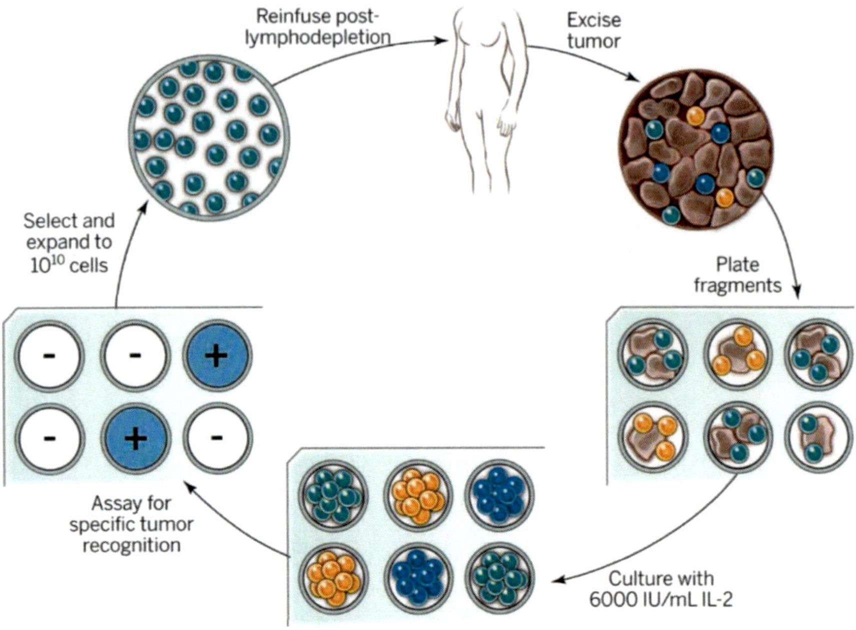

Figure 2. General schema for using the adoptive cell transfer of naturally occurring autologous tumor infiltrating lymphocytes (TILs). Reproduced with permission from Rosenberg et al. [Rosenberg SA, Restifo NP. Adoptive cell transfer as personalized immunotherapy for human cancer. Science (New York, NY). 2015;348(6230):62-8.]

Several preclinical and clinical studies have studied the regional administration of CAR-T cells including hepatic artery infusion of CAR-T cells to treat liver tumors from metastatic colorectal cancer [42]. Katz et al., further evaluated the direct intraperitoneal administration of CAR-T cells and reported superior efficacy against CEA-positive peritoneal tumors in comparison to systemically infused CAR-Ts [43]. They went on to evaluate the effects of intraperitoneal vs systemically delivered CAR-T cells against CEA in a murine model of colon adenocarcinoma. In mice receiving anti-CEA CAR-T cells intraperitoneally, a 37-fold tumor reduction was seen as compared to a three-fold decrease in tumor burden in mice receiving anti-CEA CAR-T cells by tail vein injection [43]. While intraperitoneal administration enhances regional delivery, the effectiveness of CAR-T cells in solid organ malignancies remains limited due to the immunosuppressive tumor microenvironment (TME), which restricts T-cell function by overexpression of inhibitory receptors by cells within the TME. To overcome this challenge, Katz et al., combined intraperitoneal CAR-T cell therapy with suppressor cell targeting [43]. They combined CAR-T cell treatment with depleting antibodies against myeloid-derived suppressor cells (MDSC) and regulatory T cells (Treg), which further improved efficacy against peritoneal tumors [43].

CAR-T cells may be the latest addition in the armamentarium of therapeutic strategies to manage gastric peritoneal metastasis; however, several limitations including technical issues such as the production of high numbers of CAR-T cells, and reducing their on-target/off-tumor toxicities need to be addressed prior to their clinical application. Some of these concerns are addressed by selecting specific CAR-T cell targets, such as the tumor-associated antigen mesothelin, which is frequently expressed in gastric cancer cells (NCT03608618).

T cell receptor (TCR) gene-engineered T cells are another form of adoptive T-cell therapy (ACT) that have shown promising results in the management of melanoma and synovial cell sarcoma [44]. In this form of ACT, T cells are genetically engineered by transducing TCR genes with enhanced specificity to known tumor-associated antigens [45]. However, similar to CAR-T therapy, TCR-T cells have failed to show efficacy against solid tumors partly due to the identification of a limited number of tumor-associated antigens. In a recently published study, Marcinkowski et al., described a TCR directed against Kita-Kyushu Lung Cancer Antigen-1 (KK-LC-1) [46]. KK-LC-1, encoded by the CT83 gene, is a cancer germline mutation that is highly expressed in gastric cancer. The KK-LC-1-reactive T cell receptor (KK-LC-1 TCR) was identified from the tumor-infiltrating lymphocytes (TILs) of a patient with cervical cancer. The authors reported that these genetically engineered T cells expressing KK-LC-1 TCR (KK-LC-1 TCR-Ts) demonstrated activity against CT83+ tumor lines and caused regression of CT83+ xenograft tumors in murine models [46]. Following these promising results, further clinical testing of KK-LC-1 TCR-Ts in gastric cancer is warranted.

Immunotoxin Therapy

Immunotoxin-based therapy is based on pairing bacterial exotoxin or endotoxin with an antibody conjugate that targets a protein or other marker expressed by the tumor tissue and not normal tissues [47]. This combines the specificity of the antibody of interest with the cell-killing potential of the attached toxin. An example of such an immunotoxin conjugate under clinical investigation is that of LMB-100, comprised of an anti-mesothelin Fab linked to *Pseudomonas* toxin A, with a recently completed Phase I dose-finding study [48]. Future studies of LMB-100 among gastric cancer patients whose tumors express mesothelin may provide a novel intravenous and/or intraperitoneal treatment option. Work exploring other potential immunotoxin therapies is also underway.

Cancer Vaccines

Tumor-associated antigens (TAAs) or mutation-derived antigens (neoantigens) are commonly expressed by tumor cells and can be recognized as foreign antigens, thereby eliciting both cellular and humoral immune responses. Cancer vaccines are designed to identify and target these TAAs and neoantigens in order to provoke a tumor-specific immune response. Dendritic cells (DCs), which are antigen-presenting cells capable of activating NK cells, B lymphocytes, and naïve and memory T cells, are the primary target of most cancer vaccines; however, several other effector cells such as cytotoxic T cells (CTLs) and CD4+ T-helper cells can also be targeted by several forms of cancer vaccines.

There has been much interest in developing cancer vaccines for intraperitoneal administration in peritoneal metastasis and malignant ascites associated with PM. Ai et al., evaluated the safety and efficacy of intraperitoneal injection of dendritic cell vaccines with cytokine-induced killer (CIK) cells, which are CTLs with $CD3^+$ $CD56^+$ phenotype, in patients with malignant ascites [49]. The authors reported a clinical response rate (RR) of 40.9% and a disease control rate (DCR) of 77.3%. The combination of DCs with CIK cells led to a decrease in the number of $CD4^+$ $CD25^+$ Treg cells and an increase in CTLs in ascites [49].

Virus-based immunotherapy has also been investigated as a potential treatment strategy for PM. It most commonly employs the use of oncolytic reoviruses, which are double-stranded ribonucleic acid viruses that preferentially attack and kill tumor cells. In animal models of ovarian cancer, dendritic cells, in combination with reovirus, killed ovarian cancer cells and alleviated the severity of OC, prolonging overall survival. (50) In a phase I study designed to assess the safety and antitumor activity of intraperitoneal administration of oncolytic vaccinia virus GL-ONC1 in advanced stage PM, Lauer et al., reported that GL-ONC1 was well tolerated when administered intraperitoneally and viral infection and replication were successfully established [51].

While they are a promising new development, cancer vaccines have shown inconsistent results in clinical trials and vaccine-based monotherapy is plagued with several limitations including tumor immune-evasion mechanisms and the presence of poorly immunogenic tumor antigens [52]. Consequently, there have been efforts to combine cancer vaccines with adjuvant therapies including ICI therapy or chemoradiotherapy. Cancer vaccine development will likely have to be geared towards these combinatorial regimens in the future to obtain a meaningful clinical benefit.

Nanoparticle Drug Delivery System

Despite advances in the development of systemic chemotherapeutic agents, the prognosis for gastric cancer with peritoneal disease remains poor, in part secondary to the hypothesized 'blood peritoneal barrier' that limits peritoneal penetration of intravenously administered chemotherapy [53]. Hence, attention has shifted to developing treatment strategies that have a higher potential to penetrate the peritoneum. Intraperitoneal nanoparticle drug delivery systems are considered an attractive option to maximize local drug efficacy while limiting potential systemic adverse effects.

Nano-drugs, a drug formulation measuring 20 to 100 nanometers in molecular diameter, are a promising novel drug delivery system for patients with PM. Nano-drugs are preferentially accumulated in tumor tissue as a result of either passive diffusion via the enhanced permeability and retention (EPR) effect or through the use of an active targeting moiety [54].

A pH-responsive expansile nanoparticle (eNP) drug delivery system has been designed to be administered specifically via the intraperitoneal route to treat peritoneal surface malignancies. Paclitaxel-loaded eNPs (PTX-eNPs) demonstrated increased efficacy compared to the standard clinical formulation of paclitaxel in orthotopic models of peritoneal mesothelioma and ovarian cancer, and demonstrated comparable efficacy to paclitaxel in a third model of pancreatic cancer [55]. Such eNPs can also potentially be used as a fluorescent probe to enhance visualization of peritoneal implants and assist in resection [55].

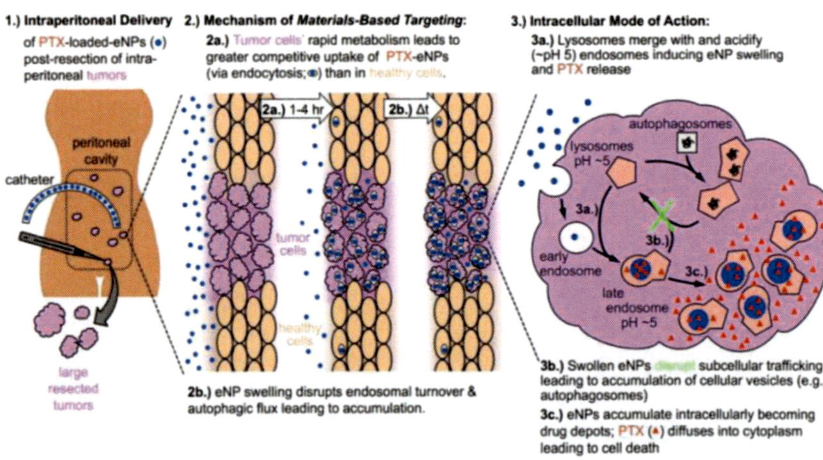

Figure 3. Schematic of expansile nanoparticle (eNP)-mediated drug delivery to peritoneal tumors. Figure reproduced with permission from Colby et al., [55].

The use of several other forms of paclitaxel-incorporating nanoparticles has been reported in the past, including NK105, which is a nanomicellar paclitaxel formulation. In one study, intraperitoneal administration of NK105 was reported to significantly reduce peritoneal disease burden compared with conventional paclitaxel formulation in a mouse model of gastric cancer [56].

Albumin has also been reported as an effective carrier for anticancer drugs that require intraperitoneal administration. Nanoparticle albumin-bound paclitaxel (nab-paclitaxel, Abraxane®), an FDA-approved drug formulation for metastatic breast cancer, was developed by Nab-technology, a patented nanotechnology-based drug delivery system. Nab-paclitaxel is a solvent-free formulation of paclitaxel that was designed to improve tumor penetration and reduce solvent-related side effects provoked by traditionally prepared solvent-based paclitaxel (sb-PTX). A phase I trial was conducted by Cristea et al., to investigate the use of intraperitoneal nab-paclitaxel in the treatment of peritoneal metastasis, and the drug was found to have a favorable toxicity profile and promising clinical activity 57]. Additionally, a comparison between the weekly administration of nab-paclitaxel (w-nab-PTX) and weekly solvent-based paclitaxel (w-sb-PTX) was conducted in the phase III ABSOLUTE trial [58]. The study reported that weekly nab-paclitaxel was non-inferior to weekly solvent-based paclitaxel in terms of overall survival and concluded that due to its improved tolerability in comparison to sb-PTX, w-nab-PTX might be a potential regimen for second-line treatment of gastric cancer. P-SELECT is an ongoing randomized phase II trial conducted by the West Japan Oncology Group that will compare w-nab-PTX to w-nab-PTX and ramucirumab in patients with unresectable advanced or recurrent gastric cancer with peritoneal dissemination that is refractory to first-line therapy [59].

Photodynamic Diagnosis and Therapy

Photodynamic diagnosis (PDD) and photodynamic therapy (PDT) have both emerged as promising avenues for the diagnosis and treatment of peritoneal metastasis. Photodynamic diagnosis utilizes photosensitizers (PS), which are agents that are capable of emitting fluorescence on excitation by visible and near-infrared light for fluorescence detection of micrometastases, whereas photodynamic therapy activates a photosensitizing agent using a specific laser wavelength and allows for the accumulation of the agent specifically at tumor sites.

PDD is a fluorescence-based optical imaging modality that most commonly utilizes 5-aminolevulinic acid (ALA) and its derivatives as photosensitizers. ALA, which is a precursor in the heme pathway, is metabolized into the potent photosensitizer protoporphyrin IX. Exogenous administration of ALA leads to a buildup of protoporphyrin IX in cancer cells. Upon excitation by specific wavelengths of light, protoporphyrin IX emits fluorescence, which in turn assists in the identification and fluorescence-guided resection of tumor cells. While PDD employs the same principle as conventional fluorescence-guided surgery, it differs in its use of photosensitizers, which can also be used for PDT. In a systematic review of 12 human and 18 animal studies evaluating PDD for diagnosis of peritoneal metastasis, PDD was found to be a safe modality, with sensitivity and specificity reported at 83%-100% and 95%-100%, respectively, in clinical studies [61]. For advanced gastric cancer, in particular, Kishi et al., evaluated PDD using 15-25 mg/kg of ALA and reported a sensitivity of 80-90% [62]. Another study investigated the diagnostic usefulness of staging fluorescence laparoscopy for gastric cancer by using 5-ALA and found it to be accurate and suitable for the detection of peritoneal metastases and of superficial liver micrometastases in patients with gastric cancer [63]. PDD does carry certain limitations as a diagnostic tool including the effect of tissue autofluorescence and insufficient depth penetration of excitation light required to activate a photosensitizer [64]. Furthermore, preoperative chemotherapy may influence the sensitivity of PDD, causing reduced uptake of ALA in residual lesions due to degeneration of the affected peritoneum caused by chemotherapeutic agents [65].

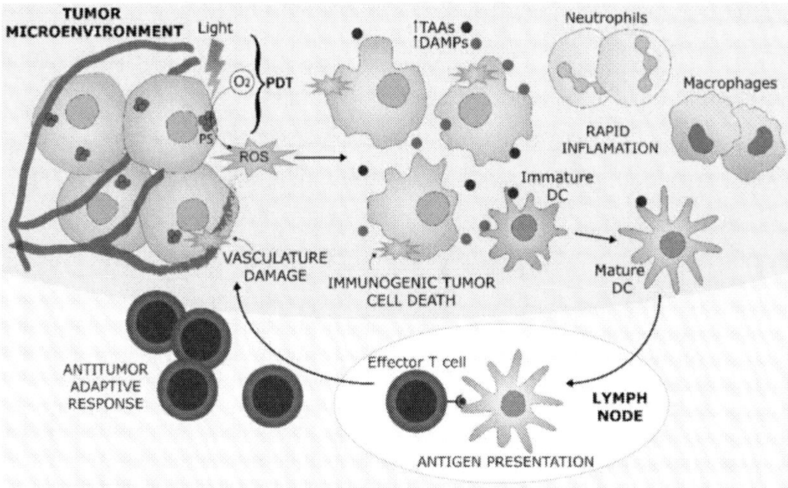

Figure 4. Overview of the antitumor mechanisms of PDT. PDT uses a photochemical reaction between a photosensitizer, light and molecular oxygen resulting in the generation of reactive oxygen species (ROS) within tumor cells and tumor-associated vasculature. Figure reproduced with permission from Beltrán Hernández et al., [60].

PDT is a clinically approved oncologic treatment strategy that employs the principle of a photochemical reaction between a photosensitizer, light, and molecular oxygen. After being administered via the intravenous or intraperitoneal route, photosensitizers preferentially accumulate in tumor cells. The exact mechanism for this preferential accumulation is unknown; however, it is hypothesized it is secondary to morphological differences in non-malignant vs tumor cells including the lack of lymphatic channels within tumor tissues [66]. PS is then activated with a particular wavelength of light, leading to a photochemical reaction resulting in reactive oxygen species (ROS) production. The interaction between ROS and oxygen causes superoxide formation which causes cytotoxicity both via a direct mechanism (autophagy, apoptosis, and necrosis) and an indirect mechanism secondary to microvascular damage. This ability of PDT to exert its effect via multiple cell death pathways allows it to be effective in even apoptosis-resistant tumor cells [61]. A systematic review of studies on the use of PDT for the treatment of peritoneal metastasis was published in 2018 and reported a significant survival advantage using PDT with CRS over CRS alone in Phase III clinical studies [61]. However, PDT has been reported to have a narrow therapeutic window and significant toxicity including capillary leak syndrome and bowel perforation [67].

PDT has also been used in combination with nanotechnology by the integration of nanoparticles with photosensitizers. This can enhance the antitumor effect of PDT by circumventing the poor cell membrane permeability and non-specificity of certain photosensitizers. Xin et al., in a study using a nano-micelle F127 integrated with a photosensitizer and novel targeting chemotherapy agent, found the combination to induce prolonged apoptosis leading to cell death in gastric cancer patients [68].

Both PDD and PDT hold promise in the management of gastric cancer peritoneal metastasis and while there is ample data from preclinical studies demonstrating the efficacy of both, there is insufficient evidence from clinical trials particularly for peritoneal metastasis, which prevents incorporation of PDD and PDT into standard clinical practice.

Cancer Gene Therapy

Cancer gene therapy involves the introduction of therapeutic genes into tumor cells to cause tumor eradication via direct and indirect mechanisms. Some of the mechanisms employed by cancer gene therapy include stimulation of a protective immune response, replacement of mutated tumor suppressor genes, inactivation of oncogenes or multidrug-resistant genes, and suicide gene therapy. Suicide gene therapy is the process of introducing a gene into a cancer cell that then encodes for an enzyme responsible for converting an anticancer prodrug to a cytotoxic drug within the cell [69, 70)]. Several vectors have been employed for the delivery of genes into cancer cells, and they can be classified into two broad categories: viral and non-viral vectors. While viral vector delivery systems have certain limitations, including the stimulation of a strong immune response against the proteinaceous capsid of a virus, most clinical trials on cancer gene therapy employ the use of viral vector-based delivery systems. Adenoviruses are the most commonly used viral vectors because of their ability to infect a broad range of cell types and the ease with which their genome can be manipulated make them ideal vector candidates [71]. In non-viral vector delivery systems, nanoparticle-mediated delivery of suicide genes has been found to be an effective method [72]. Carruthers et al., developed a gene-directed enzyme pro-drug therapy (GDEPT) system in which the gene encoding an enzyme involved in drug metabolism is delivered to tumor cells, followed by administration of a pro-drug, to ensure localized drug delivery of a potentially toxic chemotherapeutic agent. They used recombinant adeno-associated virus (rAAV) to deliver β-galactosidase (LacZ) to a treatment group and green fluorescent protein to a control group. Adenocarcinoma cells were then injected at the same site as the rAAV in both groups after a week. An hour later, the pro-drug geldanamycin was intraperitoneally injected. Tumor growth was found to be significantly suppressed in animals who received the β-galactosidase gene [73].

Several pre-clinical studies have evaluated the role of gene therapy in peritoneal metastasis. In a study investigating the efficacy of combined suicide and cytokine gene therapy in a model of colorectal peritoneal metastasis in syngeneic rats, Lechanteur et al., reported significantly improved survival in animals treated with a suicide gene (herpes simplex virus type I thymidine kinase (HSV-TK)) and cytokine genes [74]. In another study, an adenoviral construct of the human p14ARF tumor suppressor gene (Ad-hARF) was administered into a mouse model of peritoneal metastasis derived from human colorectal cancer cell line (Clone A) cells. A single intraperitoneal dose of Ad-hARF suppressed the progression of peritoneal disease, and the same result was seen with weekly administration for six weeks [75].

Gene transfer technology in cancer therapy has been rapidly evolving, but its feasibility and efficacy for peritoneal metastasis have not as of yet been demonstrated in clinical trials. Future developments in the field of cancer gene therapy will hopefully lead to more robust evidence of its application in the management of peritoneal metastasis.

Near-Infrared Photoimmunotherapy

Near-infrared photoimmunotherapy (NIR-PIT) is a molecularly targeted phototherapy that uses an antibody-photo-absorber conjugate (APC) that is activated by ncar-infrared light. It involves injecting a conjugate of a near-infrared, water-soluble dye IRdye700DX (IR700), and a monoclonal antibody (mAb) directed against cancer cell surface markers. NIR-PIT works on the principle that near-infrared light can kill cancer cells that have membrane-bound mAb conjugates (trastuzumab and panitumumab) of the NIR activatable IR700 dye leading to highly selective immunogenic cell death while non-cell surface-bound conjugates had no effect [76, 77].

Researchers at the National Cancer Institute, National Institutes of Health in Maryland, USA evaluated the efficacy of endoscopic NIR-PIT using a fiberoptic diffuser for peritoneal metastasis in gastric cancer in a mouse model. They applied NIR-PIT using an APC trastuzumab-IR700DX (tra-IR700) in human epidermal growth factor 2 positive (HER2+) gastric carcinoma and found high tumor accumulation of tra-IR700 within peritoneal implants on fluorescence endoscopy. The endoscopic NIR-PIT group had a significantly greater therapeutic effect compared to the control groups. Moreover, histopathological analysis showed diffuse cancer cell death in NIR-PIT-treated tumors [78].

NIR-PIT differs in principle from PDT and carries significant advantages over PDT since the hydrophobic nature of the porphyrin photosensitizers used in PDT makes them difficult to target, leading to reduced selectivity and thereby causing more toxicity. NIR-PIT technology could have much wider application once mAbs targeting other cell surface markers can be developed and used as APC in malignancies with different molecular signatures.

Cell-Free and Concentrated Ascites Reinfusion Therapy (CART)

Originally developed for the management of ascites in cirrhotic patients, cell-free and concentrated ascites reinfusion therapy is one of the types of apheresis treatments, by which filtered and concentrated ascites containing albumin and globulin is reinfused intravenously to patients. Massive malignant ascites originating from peritoneal metastasis of gastric cancer is difficult to control and is frequently resistant to both IV and IP chemotherapy. CART has been proven to be effective in the palliative management of massive ascites in patients with gastric PM. Ito et al., studied the effect of CART on symptom relief in patients with malignant ascites and found that all 37 patients in the study experienced symptom relief within 24 hours of CART [79]. Furthermore, combining CART with intraperitoneal paclitaxel administration has enabled patients with massive ascites to receive intraperitoneal chemotherapy with improved survival [80, 81].

The Future Perspective – Tissue Models of Peritoneal Metastasis from Gastric Cancer and Ongoing Clinical Research

Several tissue model systems of gastric cancer and peritoneal metastasis that are designed to mimic the pathophysiological features of human tissue are currently employed in basic science and translational research. Murine models are perhaps the most widely used experimental models. Imano et al., created a novel animal model of peritoneal metastasis by injecting colonic adenocarcinoma cell line RCN-9 subcutaneously or into the cecal subserosa of Fisher 344 rats. This model was an improvement from previous animal models in which cancer cells did not coat the peritoneum like tumors but instead formed discrete tumor nodules in the omentum, liver hilum, mesentery, diaphragm, and the subcutaneous tissue [82]. Mei et al., created the first large animal model of peritoneal metastasis from gastric cancer by laparotomic orthotopic injection of VX2 cancer cells into the submucosal layer of the stomach in rabbits. They then went on to evaluate therapeutic cytoreductive surgery (CRS) with or without hyperthermic intraperitoneal chemotherapy (HIPEC) in their model and reported CRS alone could not bring benefit while CRS + HIPEC with docetaxel and carboplatin could significantly prolong survival [83].

Four different types of xenograft mouse models of peritoneal dissemination of gastric cancer were created by Okazaki and colleagues [84]. In a study conducted to demonstrate the contribution of human peritoneal mesothelial cells (HPMCs) to fibrotic tumor formation, the authors developed a new xenograft model of peritoneal metastasis that can be used to analyze the pathophysiology of peritoneal dissemination of gastric cancer.

Organoids have also served as effective pre-clinical models for gastric cancer. Yan et al., established a biobank of patient-derived gastric cancer organoids that include a wide range of gastric cancer molecular subtypes. Moreover, they found these organoids maintained long-term similarity to the original tumors and were suitable for targeted drug testing [85)]. Malignant ascites-derived organoid (MADO) cultures for gastric cancer have also been established for in vitro modeling and targeted drug evaluation [86].

Investigators at the National Institutes of Health, Maryland, USA have created a novel ex-vivo perfusion circuit, the SMART (**S**urgically resected tu**M**or with int**A**ct microenvi**R**onmen**T**) system that sustains tumor-bearing human peritoneum affixed to platforms in a perfusion circuit for up to seven days [87]. This approach preserves tumor nodule deposits with their intact microenvironment. The SMART system not only allows for interrogation with immunomodulatory agents and targeted drugs but is also amenable to three-dimensional live-cell imaging and endpoint analysis of identical samples by immunohistochemistry and *in situ* RNA analysis. This system has unique translational applicability and serves as the next step in personalized cancer therapy.

At present, several clinical trials are investigating the role of CRS in combination with different regimens of adjuvant chemotherapy in gastric peritoneal metastasis. A study being conducted at the National Taiwan University Hospital, Taiwan [Clinicaltrials.gov Identifier: NCT04547725] is evaluating the 6-month disease control rate (DCR) of complete CRS combined with normothermic intraperitoneal chemotherapy (N-IPEC) and systemic chemotherapy for gastric adenocarcinoma with limited PM. The trial will be carried out in two stages with a total number of 13 patients accrued in the first stage. If there are ≤6 progression-free patients, the study will be stopped. Otherwise, an additional 17 patients will be accrued in stage II, resulting in a total sample size of 30. All patients will undergo a D2 gastrectomy and complete CRS followed by N-IPEC with paclitaxel and systemic chemotherapy (high-dose fluorouracil and cisplatin [P-HDFL], or capecitabine and oxaliplatin [CAPOX]). A ≥75% 6-month DCR is expected to be achieved.

Multiple clinical trials are assessing the combination of intraperitoneal paclitaxel with various systemic chemotherapeutic regimens. In a phase I/II trial, researchers at the Seoul National University Bundang Hospital, South Korea, are studying the combination of intraperitoneal chemotherapy (Paclitaxel) + systemic mFOLFOX6(5-FU, Oxaliplatin, Leucovorin) regimen. The primary outcome measures will be dose determination (phase I) and 1-year overall survival (phase 2) [ClinicalTrials.gov Identifier: NCT03618758]. Another phase II nonrandomized study aims to determine progression-free survival (PFS) in patients with gastric peritoneal metastasis after repeated intraperitoneal chemotherapeutic infusion (IPC) and systemic paclitaxel administration with concomitant capecitabine therapy [ClinicalTrials.gov Identifier: NCT04034251].

The efficacy of HIPEC combined with systemic chemotherapy and CRS in the treatment of PM from gastric cancer is being evaluated in a multicenter phase III randomized study in China. Patients will be divided into two arms: experimental and control groups. In the experimental arm, patients will receive HIPEC, followed by NACT, CRS, HIPEC, and finally adjuvant chemotherapy. In the control group, patients will receive neoadjuvant chemotherapy followed by CRS and adjuvant chemotherapy.

The primary outcome measure will median overall survival for 3 years [ClinicalTrials.gov Identifier: NCT03179579]. A multicenter phase I / II trial in France is determining the maximal tolerated dose (MTD) with dose escalation of oxaliplatin via a laparoscopic approach of aerosol pressurized intraperitoneal chemotherapy (PIPAC) for nonresectable peritoneal disease from digestive cancers, including gastric cancer [ClinicalTrials.gov Identifier: NCT03294252].

The Dragon II trial is a multicenter phase III randomized controlled trial that is studying the efficiency of the combination of neoadjuvant chemotherapy (NAC) and neoadjuvant laparoscopic intraperitoneal hyperthermic chemotherapy (NLHIPEC) followed by R0 gastrectomy with intraoperative HIPEC for advanced gastric cancer. This trial will be the first to study the combination of NAC and NLHIPEC in the preoperative setting. A total of 326 patients will be randomly divided into 2 groups in a 1:1 ratio after laparoscopic exploration. The control group will undergo standard R0 D2 gastrectomy followed by 8 cycles of adjuvant chemotherapy with oxaliplatin with S-1 (SOX) regimen while the experiment group will receive the proposed Dragon II regimen. Per study protocol, the combination of NLHIPEC with NAC and HIPEC will increase progression-free survival (PFS) by 15% [88].

CONCLUSION

With significant advances in the management of peritoneal metastasis in the last decade, it is no longer considered an imminent death sentence. However, when it comes to PM in gastric cancer, there still is a lack of a standardized treatment strategy that reliably leads to significantly improved survival. The constantly evolving novel intraperitoneal therapeutic options for PM need to be further evaluated in clinical trials to develop individualized treatment strategies that improve the prognosis of this dismal disease.

REFERENCES

[1] Ji L, Selleck MJ, Morgan JW, Xu J, Babcock BD, Shavlik D, et al., Gastric Cancer Peritoneal Carcinomatosis Risk Score. *Ann Surg Oncol.* 2020;27(1):240-7.

[2] Wang R, Song S, Harada K, Ghazanfari Amlashi F, Badgwell B, Pizzi MP, et al., Multiplex profiling of peritoneal metastases from gastric adenocarcinoma identified novel targets and molecular subtypes that predict treatment response. *Gut.* 2020;69(1):18-31.

[3] Qu L, He L, Jia Z, Wang Q. Prognostic value of CEA/CA72-4 immunohistochemistry in combination with cytology for detecting tumor cells in peritoneal lavage in gastric cancer. *Journal of Cancer.* 2020;11(21):6319-25.

[4] Nakanishi H, Kodera Y, Yamamura Y, Ito S, Kato T, Ezaki T, et al., Rapid quantitative detection of carcinoembryonic antigen-expressing free tumor cells in the peritoneal cavity of gastric-cancer patients with real-time RT-PCR on the lightcycler. *International journal of cancer.* 2000;89(5):411-7.

[5] Dalal KM, Woo Y, Kelly K, Galanis C, Gonen M, Fong Y, et al., Detection of micrometastases in peritoneal washings of gastric cancer patients by the reverse transcriptase polymerase chain reaction. *Gastric cancer: official journal of the International Gastric Cancer Association and the Japanese Gastric Cancer Association.* 2008;11(4):206-13.

[6] Yamamoto M, Baba H, Kakeji Y, Endo K, Ikeda Y, Toh Y, et al., Prognostic significance of tumor markers in peritoneal lavage in advanced gastric cancer. *Oncology.* 2004;67(1):19-26.

[7] Kodera Y, Nakanishi H, Ito S, Yamamura Y, Fujiwara M, Koike M, et al., Prognostic significance of intraperitoneal cancer cells in gastric carcinoma: detection of cytokeratin 20 mRNA in peritoneal washes, in addition to detection of carcinoembryonic antigen. Gastric cancer: *official journal of the International Gastric Cancer Association and the Japanese Gastric Cancer Association.* 2005;8(3):142-8.

[8] Lorenzen S, Panzram B, Rosenberg R, Nekarda H, Becker K, Schenk U, et al., Prognostic significance of free peritoneal tumor cells in the peritoneal cavity before and after neoadjuvant chemotherapy in patients with gastric carcinoma undergoing potentially curative resection. *Ann Surg Oncol.* 2010;17(10):2733-9.

[9] Nekarda H, Gess C, Stark M, Mueller JD, Fink U, Schenck U, et al., Immunocytochemically detected free peritoneal tumour cells (FPTC) are a strong prognostic factor in gastric carcinoma. *British journal of cancer.* 1999;79(3-4):611-9.

[10] Rosenberg R, Nekarda H, Bauer P, Schenck U, Hoefler H, Siewert JR. Free peritoneal tumour cells are an independent prognostic factor in curatively resected stage IB gastric carcinoma. *The British journal of surgery.* 2006;93(3):325-31.

[11] Li Z, Zhang D, Zhang H, Miao Z, Tang Y, Sun G, et al., Prediction of peritoneal recurrence by the mRNA level of CEA and MMP-7 in peritoneal lavage of gastric cancer patients. Tumour biology: *the journal of the International Society for Oncodevelopmental Biology and Medicine.* 2014;35(4):3463-70.

[12] Yonemura Y, Fujimura T, Ninomiya I, Kim BS, Bandou E, Sawa T, et al., Prediction of peritoneal micrometastasis by peritoneal lavaged cytology and reverse transcriptase-polymerase chain reaction for matrix metalloproteinase-7 mRNA. Clinical cancer research: *an official journal of the American Association for Cancer Research.* 2001;7(6):1647-53.

[13] Iida T, Iwahashi M, Katsuda M, Ishida K, Nakamori M, Nakamura M, et al., Prognostic significance of IL-17 mRNA expression in peritoneal lavage in gastric cancer patients who underwent curative resection. *Oncology reports.* 2014;31(2):605-12.

[14] Mori K, Suzuki T, Uozaki H, Nakanishi H, Ueda T, Matsuno Y, et al., Detection of minimal gastric cancer cells in peritoneal washings by focused microarray analysis with multiple markers: clinical implications. *Ann Surg Oncol.* 2007;14(5):1694-702.

[15] Chen Y, Zhou Q, Wang H, Zhuo W, Ding Y, Lu J, et al., Predicting Peritoneal Dissemination of Gastric Cancer in the Era of Precision

Medicine: Molecular Characterization and Biomarkers. *Cancers.* 2020;12(8).

[16] Ohzawa H, Saito A, Kumagai Y, Kimura Y, Yamaguchi H, Hosoya Y, et al., Reduced expression of exosomal miR-29s in peritoneal fluid is a useful predictor of peritoneal recurrence after curative resection of gastric cancer with serosal involvement. *Oncology* reports. 2020;43(4):1081-8.

[17] Baumgartner JM, Riviere P, Lanman RB, Kelly KJ, Veerapong J, Lowy AM, et al., Prognostic Utility of Pre- and Postoperative Circulating Tumor DNA Liquid Biopsies in Patients with Peritoneal Metastases. *Ann Surg Oncol.* 2020;27(9):3259-67.

[18] Soeda N, Iinuma H, Suzuki Y, Tsukahara D, Midorikawa H, Igarashi Y, et al., Plasma exosome-encapsulated microRNA-21 and microRNA-92a are promising biomarkers for the prediction of peritoneal recurrence in patients with gastric cancer. *Oncology letters.* 2019;18(5):4467-80.

[19] Kim M, Jeong WK, Lim S, Sohn TS, Bae JM, Sohn IS. Gastric cancer: development and validation of a CT-based model to predict peritoneal metastasis. Acta radiologica (Stockholm, *Sweden*: 1987). 2020;61(6):732-42.

[20] Liu S, He J, Liu S, Ji C, Guan W, Chen L, et al., Radiomics analysis using contrast-enhanced CT for preoperative prediction of occult peritoneal metastasis in advanced gastric cancer. *European radiology*. 2020;30(1):239-46.

[21] Huang Z, Liu D, Chen X, Yu P, Wu J, Song B, et al., Retrospective imaging studies of gastric cancer: Study protocol clinical trial (SPIRIT Compliant). *Medicine.* 2020;99(8):e19157.

[22] Hoogstins CE, Weixler B, Boogerd LS, Hoppener DJ, Prevoo HA, Sier CF, et al., In Search for Optimal Targets for Intraoperative Fluorescence Imaging of Peritoneal Metastasis From Colorectal Cancer. *Biomarkers in cancer.* 2017;9:1179299x17728254.

[23] Fujita T, Seshimo A, Kameoka S. Detection of sentinel nodes in gastric cancer by indocyanine green fluorescence imaging. *Hepato-gastroenterology*. 2012;59(119):2213-6.

[24] Okubo K, Uenosono Y, Arigami T, Matsushita D, Yanagita S, Kijima T, et al., Quantitative assessment of fluorescence intensity of ICG in sentinel nodes in early gastric cancer. Gastric cancer: *official journal of the International Gastric Cancer Association and the Japanese Gastric Cancer Association.* 2018;21(5):776-81.

[25] Baiocchi GL, Gheza F, Molfino S, Arru L, Vaira M, Giacopuzzi S. Indocyanine green fluorescence-guided intraoperative detection of peritoneal carcinomatosis: systematic review. *BMC Surgery.* 2020;20(1):158.

[26] Maubert A, Birtwisle L, Bernard JL, Benizri E, Bereder JM. Can machine learning predict resecability of a peritoneal carcinomatosis? *Surgical oncology*. 2019;29:120-5.

[27] Chua YJ, Cunningham D. The UK NCRI MAGIC Trial of Perioperative Chemotherapy in Resectable Gastric Cancer: Implications for Clinical Practice. *Annals of Surgical Oncology.* 2007;14(10):2687-90.

[28] Schulz C, Kullmann F, Kunzmann V, Fuchs M, Geissler M, Vehling-Kaiser U, et al., NeoFLOT: Multicenter phase II study of perioperative chemotherapy in resectable adenocarcinoma of the gastroesophageal junction or gastric adenocarcinoma-Very good response predominantly in patients with intestinal type tumors. *International journal of cancer.* 2015;137(3):678-85.

[29] Ganschow P, Hofmann L, Stintzing S, Heinemann V, Angele M, Werner J, et al., Operative Results and Perioperative Morbidity After Intensified Neoadjuvant Chemotherapy with FLOT for Gastroesophageal Adenocarcinoma Impact of Intensified Neoadjuvant Treatment. Journal of gastrointestinal surgery : *official journal of the Society for Surgery of the Alimentary Tract.* 2020.

[30] Roeland E, Kanter K, Wo JYL, Fish M, Nipp RD, Seventer EEV, et al., Preliminary analysis of total neoadjuvant therapy for patients with locally advanced gastric (G) and gastroesophageal (GE) adenocarcinoma. 2020;38(4_suppl):393-.

[31] Greally M, Strong VE, Yoon SS, Coit DG, Chou JF, Capanu M, et al., Total neoadjuvant chemo (ctx; TNT) for locally advanced gastric

cancer (GC): *The Memorial Sloan Kettering Cancer Center experience.* 2019;37(15_suppl):4046-.

[32] Zappasodi R, Merghoub T, Wolchok JD. Emerging Concepts for Immune Checkpoint Blockade-Based Combination Therapies. *Cancer cell.* 2018;33(4):581-98.

[33] Fuchs CS, Doi T, Jang RW, Muro K, Satoh T, Machado M, et al., Safety and Efficacy of Pembrolizumab Monotherapy in Patients With Previously Treated Advanced Gastric and Gastroesophageal Junction Cancer: Phase 2 Clinical KEYNOTE-059 Trial. *JAMA oncology.* 2018;4(5):e180013.

[34] Katz H, Biglow L, Alsharedi M. Immune Checkpoint Inhibitors in Locally Advanced, Unresectable, and Metastatic Upper Gastrointestinal Malignancies. *Journal of gastrointestinal cancer.* 2020;51(2):611-9.

[35] Rotte A, Jin JY, Lemaire V. Mechanistic overview of immune checkpoints to support the rational design of their combinations in cancer immunotherapy. Annals of oncology: *official journal of the European Society for Medical Oncology.* 2018;29(1):71-83.

[36] Figueroa-Protti L, Soto-Molinari R, Calderón-Osorno M, Mora J, Alpízar-Alpízar W. Gastric Cancer in the Era of Immune Checkpoint Blockade. *Journal of oncology.* 2019;2019:1079710.

[37] Ströhlein MA, Heiss MM, Jauch KW. The current status of immunotherapy in peritoneal carcinomatosis. *Expert review of anticancer therapy.* 2016;16(10):1019-27.

[38] Heiss MM, Ströhlein MA, Jäger M, Kimmig R, Burges A, Schoberth A, et al., Immunotherapy of malignant ascites with trifunctional antibodies. *International journal of cancer.* 2005;117(3):435-43.

[39] Heiss MM, Murawa P, Koralewski P, Kutarska E, Kolesnik OO, Ivanchenko VV, et al., The trifunctional antibody catumaxomab for the treatment of malignant ascites due to epithelial cancer: Results of a prospective randomized phase II/III trial. *International journal of cancer.* 2010;127(9):2209-21.

[40] Thadi A, Khalili M, Morano WF, Richard SD, Katz SC, Bowne WB. Early Investigations and Recent Advances in Intraperitoneal Immunotherapy for Peritoneal Metastasis. *Vaccines.* 2018;6(3).

[41] Bębnowska D, Grywalska E, Niedźwiedzka-Rystwej P, Sosnowska-Pasiarska B, Smok-Kalwat J, Pasiarski M, et al., CAR-T Cell Therapy-An Overview of Targets in Gastric Cancer. *Journal of clinical medicine.* 2020;9(6).

[42] Katz SC, Burga RA, McCormack E, Wang LJ, Mooring W, Point GR, et al., Phase I Hepatic Immunotherapy for Metastases Study of Intra-Arterial Chimeric Antigen Receptor-Modified T-cell Therapy for CEA+ Liver Metastases. *Clinical cancer research: an official journal of the American Association for Cancer Research.* 2015;21(14):3149-59.

[43] Katz SC, Point GR, Cunetta M, Thorn M, Guha P, Espat NJ, et al., Regional CAR-T cell infusions for peritoneal carcinomatosis are superior to systemic delivery. *Cancer gene therapy.* 2016;23(5):142-8.

[44] Robbins PF, Kassim SH, Tran TL, Crystal JS, Morgan RA, Feldman SA, et al., A pilot trial using lymphocytes genetically engineered with an NY-ESO-1-reactive T-cell receptor: long-term follow-up and correlates with response. *Clinical cancer research: an official journal of the American Association for Cancer Research.* 2015;21(5):1019-27.

[45] Li D, Li X, Zhou WL, Huang Y, Liang X, Jiang L, et al., Genetically engineered T cells for cancer immunotherapy. *Signal Transduction and Targeted Therapy.* 2019;4(1):35.

[46] Marcinkowski B, Stevanović S, Helman SR, Norberg SM, Serna C, Jin B, et al., Cancer targeting by TCR gene-engineered T cells directed against Kita-Kyushu Lung Cancer Antigen-1. *Journal for ImmunoTherapy of Cancer.* 2019;7(1):229.

[47] Pastan I, Hassan R, Fitzgerald DJ, Kreitman RJ. Immunotoxin therapy of cancer. *Nature reviews Cancer.* 2006;6(7):559-65.

[48] Hassan R, Alewine C, Mian I, Spreafico A, Siu LL, Gomez-Roca C, et al., Phase 1 study of the immunotoxin LMB-100 in patients with

mesothelioma and other solid tumors expressing mesothelin. *Cancer.* 2020;126(22):4936-47.

[49] Ai YQ, Cai K, Hu JH, Jiang LW, Gao YR, Zhao H, et al., The clinical effects of dendritic cell vaccines combined with cytokine-induced killer cells intraperitoneal injected on patients with malignant ascites. *International journal of clinical and experimental medicine.* 2014;7(11):4272-81.

[50] Gujar S, Dielschneider R, Clements D, Helson E, Shmulevitz M, Marcato P, et al., Multifaceted therapeutic targeting of ovarian peritoneal carcinomatosis through virus-induced immunomodulation. Molecular therapy : *the journal of the American Society of Gene Therapy.* 2013;21(2):338-47.

[51] Lauer UM, Schell M, Beil J, Berchtold S, Koppenhöfer U, Glatzle J, et al., Phase I Study of Oncolytic Vaccinia Virus GL-ONC1 in Patients with Peritoneal Carcinomatosis. *Clinical cancer research*: *an official journal of the American Association for Cancer Research.* 2018;24(18):4388-98.

[52] Bowen WS, Svrivastava AK, Batra L, Barsoumian H, Shirwan H. Current challenges for cancer vaccine adjuvant development. *Expert review of vaccines.* 2018;17(3):207-15.

[53] Dedrick RL, Flessner MF. Pharmacokinetic Problems in Peritoneal Drug Administration: Tissue Penetration and Surface Exposure. *JNCI: Journal of the National Cancer Institute.* 1997;89(7):480-7.

[54] Salvioni L, Rizzuto MA, Bertolini JA, Pandolfi L, Colombo M, Prosperi D. Thirty Years of Cancer Nanomedicine: Success, Frustration, and Hope. *Cancers.* 2019;11(12).

[55] Colby AH, Oberlies NH, Pearce CJ, Herrera VL, Colson YL, Grinstaff MW. Nanoparticle drug-delivery systems for peritoneal cancers: a case study of the design, characterization and development of the expansile nanoparticle. *Wiley interdisciplinary reviews Nanomedicine and nanobiotechnology*. 2017;9(3).

[56] Emoto S, Yamaguchi H, Kishikawa J, Yamashita H, Ishigami H, Kitayama J. Antitumor effect and pharmacokinetics of intraperitoneal

NK105, a nanomicellar paclitaxel formulation for peritoneal dissemination. *Cancer science.* 2012;103(7):1304-10.

[57] Cristea MC, Frankel P, Synold T, Rivkin S, Lim D, Chung V, et al., A phase I trial of intraperitoneal nab-paclitaxel in the treatment of advanced malignancies primarily confined to the peritoneal cavity. *Cancer chemotherapy and pharmacology.* 2019;83(3):589-98.

[58] Shitara K, Takashima A, Fujitani K, Koeda K, Hara H, Nakayama N, et al., Nab-paclitaxel versus solvent-based paclitaxel in patients with previously treated advanced gastric cancer (ABSOLUTE): an open-label, randomised, non-inferiority, phase 3 trial. *The lancet Gastroenterology & hepatology.* 2017;2(4):277-87.

[59] Hirata K, Hamamoto Y, Ando M, Imamura CK, Yoshimura K, Yamazaki K, et al., Weekly paclitaxel plus ramucirumab versus weekly nab-paclitaxel plus ramucirumab for unresectable advanced or recurrent gastric cancer with peritoneal dissemination refractory to first-line therapy-the P-SELECT trial (WJOG10617G)-a randomised phase II trial by the West Japan Oncology Group. *BMC cancer.* 2020;20(1):548.

[60] Beltrán Hernández I, Yu Y, Ossendorp F, Korbelik M, Oliveira S. Preclinical and Clinical Evidence of Immune Responses Triggered in Oncologic Photodynamic Therapy: Clinical Recommendations. *Journal of clinical medicine.* 2020;9(2).

[61] Pinto A, Pocard M. Photodynamic therapy and photothermal therapy for the treatment of peritoneal metastasis: a systematic review. *Pleura and peritoneum.* 2018;3(4):20180124.

[62] Kishi K, Fujiwara Y, Yano M, Motoori M, Sugimura K, Takahashi H, et al., Usefulness of diagnostic laparoscopy with 5-aminolevulinic acid (ALA)-mediated photodynamic diagnosis for the detection of peritoneal micrometastasis in advanced gastric cancer after chemotherapy. *Surgery today.* 2016;46(12):1427-34.

[63] Murayama Y, Ichikawa D, Koizumi N, Komatsu S, Shiozaki A, Kuriu Y, et al., Staging fluorescence laparoscopy for gastric cancer by using 5-aminolevulinic acid. *Anticancer research.* 2012;32(12):5421-7.

[64] Koizumi N, Harada Y, Minamikawa T, Tanaka H, Otsuji E, Takamatsu T. Recent advances in photodynamic diagnosis of gastric cancer using 5-aminolevulinic acid. *World journal of gastroenterology*. 2016;22(3):1289-96.

[65] Xu S, Bulin AL, Hurbin A, Elleaume H, Coll JL, Broekgaarden M. Photodynamic Diagnosis and Therapy for Peritoneal Carcinomatosis: Emerging Perspectives. *Cancers*. 2020;12(9).

[66] van Straten D, Mashayekhi V, de Bruijn HS, Oliveira S, Robinson DJ. Oncologic Photodynamic Therapy: Basic Principles, Current Clinical Status and Future Directions. *Cancers*. 2017;9(2).

[67] Almerie MQ, Gossedge G, Wright KE, Jayne DG. Treatment of peritoneal carcinomatosis with photodynamic therapy: Systematic review of current evidence. *Photodiagnosis and photodynamic therapy*. 2017;20:276-86.

[68] Xin J, Wang S, Wang J, Wang J, Fu L, Shen L, et al., Nanosystem Integrated with Photosensitizer and Novel Targeting Chemotherapy Agent for Gastric Cancer Chemo-Photodynamic Combined Therapy. *Journal of biomedical nanotechnology*. 2018;14(8):1430-47.

[69] Hallaj-Nezhadi S, Dass CR, Lotfipour F. Intraperitoneal delivery of nanoparticles for cancer gene therapy. *Future oncology* (London, England). 2013;9(1):59-68.

[70] Nezhadi SH, Choong PF, Lotfipour F, Dass CR. Gelatin-based delivery systems for cancer gene therapy. *Journal of drug targeting*. 2009;17(10):731-8.

[71] Khalighinejad N, Hariri H, Behnamfar O, Yousefi A, Momeni A. Adenoviral gene therapy in gastric cancer: a review. *World journal of gastroenterology*. 2008;14(2):180-4.

[72] Vago R, Collico V, Zuppone S, Prosperi D, Colombo M. Nanoparticle-mediated delivery of suicide genes in cancer therapy. *Pharmacological research*. 2016;111:619-41.

[73] Carruthers KH, Metzger G, During MJ, Muravlev A, Wang C, Kocak E. Gene-directed enzyme prodrug therapy for localized chemotherapeutics in allograft and xenograft tumor models. *Cancer gene therapy*. 2014;21(10):434-40.

[74] Lechanteur C, Delvenne P, Princen F, Lopez M, Fillet G, Gielen J, et al., Combined suicide and cytokine gene therapy for peritoneal carcinomatosis. *Gut.* 2000;47(3):343-8.

[75] Rajeshkumar BR, Paliwal S, Lambert L, Grossman SR, Whalen GF. Treatment of peritoneal carcinomatosis with intraperitoneal administration of Ad-hARF. *The Journal of surgical research.* 2015;197(1):85-90.

[76] Kobayashi H, Griffiths GL, Choyke PL. Near-Infrared Photoimmunotherapy: Photoactivatable Antibody-Drug Conjugates (ADCs). *Bioconjugate chemistry.* 2020;31(1):28-36.

[77] Kobayashi H, Choyke PL. Near-Infrared Photoimmunotherapy of Cancer. *Accounts of chemical research.* 2019;52(8):2332-9.

[78] Nagaya T, Okuyama S, Ogata F, Maruoka Y, Choyke PL, Kobayashi H. Endoscopic near infrared photoimmunotherapy using a fiber optic diffuser for peritoneal dissemination of gastric cancer. *Cancer science.* 2018;109(6):1902-8.

[79] Ito T, Hanafusa N, Iwase S, Noiri E, Nangaku M, Nakagawa K, et al., Effects of cell-free and concentrated ascites reinfusion therapy (CART) on symptom relief of malignancy-related ascites. *International journal of clinical oncology.* 2015;20(3):623-8.

[80] Kitayama J, Ishigami H, Yamaguchi H, Sakuma Y, Horie H, Hosoya Y, et al., Treatment of patients with peritoneal metastases from gastric cancer. *Annals of gastroenterological surgery.* 2018;2(2):116-23.

[81] Yamaguchi H, Kitayama J, Emoto S, Ishigami H, Ito T, Hanafusa N, et al., Cell-free and concentrated ascites reinfusion therapy (CART) for management of massive malignant ascites in gastric cancer patients with peritoneal metastasis treated with intravenous and intraperitoneal paclitaxel with oral S-1. European journal of surgical oncology : *the journal of the European Society of Surgical Oncology and the British Association of Surgical Oncology.* 2015;41(7):875-80.

[82] Imano M, Itoh T, Satou T, Kido A, Tsubaki M, Yasuda A, et al., Establishment of a novel model of peritoneal carcinomatosis of the peritoneal extension type. *Anticancer research.* 2013;33(4):1439-46.

[83] Tang L, Mei LJ, Yang XJ, Huang CQ, Zhou YF, Yonemura Y, et al., Cytoreductive surgery plus hyperthermic intraperitoneal chemotherapy improves survival of gastric cancer with peritoneal carcinomatosis: evidence from an experimental study. *Journal of translational medicine.* 2011;9:53.

[84] Okazaki M, Fushida S, Harada S, Tsukada T, Kinoshita J, Oyama K, et al., Establishing a xenograft mouse model of peritoneal dissemination of gastric cancer with organ invasion and fibrosis. *BMC cancer.* 2017;17(1):23.

[85] Yan HHN, Siu HC, Law S, Ho SL, Yue SSK, Tsui WY, et al., A Comprehensive Human Gastric Cancer Organoid Biobank Captures Tumor Subtype Heterogeneity and Enables Therapeutic Screening. *Cell stem cell.* 2018;23(6):882-97.e11.

[86] Li J, Xu H, Zhang L, Song L, Feng D, Peng X, et al., Malignant ascites-derived organoid (MADO) cultures for gastric cancer in vitro modelling and drug screening. *Journal of cancer research and clinical oncology.* 2019;145(11):2637-47.

[87] JM H. *SMART (Sample Microenvironment from Resected Metastatic Tumors) Platform.* U.S. Application No. 62/988,783, filed March 2020. Patent pending.

[88] Beeharry MK, Ni ZT, Yang ZY, Zheng YN, Feng RH, Liu WT, et al., Study protocol of a multicenter phase III randomized controlled trial investigating the efficiency of the combination of neoadjuvant chemotherapy (NAC) and neoadjuvant laparoscopic intraperitoneal hyperthermic chemotherapy (NLHIPEC) followed by R0 gastrectomy with intraoperative HIPEC for advanced gastric cancer (AGC): dragon II trial. *BMC cancer.* 2020;20(1):224.

About the Editors

Fernando López, MD, PhD

Chief of Upper Gastrointestinal and Peritoneal Oncology Surgery Unit, Hospital Clínico Universitario, Valencia, Spain
Associate Professor, Department of Surgery, University of Valencia

More than 25 years performing Upper gastrointestinal surgery, especially cancer cases. Associate Professor of the Department of Surgery (University of Valencia) for 10 years. Editor of 1 book on esophageal cancer (Nova Publishers). More than 10 book chapters and more than 50 peer-reviewed articles published

Roberto Martí, MD, PhD

Staff surgeon Upper Gastrointestinal and Peritoneal Oncology Surgery Unit, Hospital Clínico Universitario, Valencia, Spain

More than 25 years performing Upper gastrointestinal surgery, especially cancer cases. Co-editor of a book on esophageal cancer. Many book chapters and article published. He was associate professor in the Department of Surgery at University of Valencia

INDEX

C

D

E

F

G

H

I

J

K

L

M

N

O

P

Q

R

S

T

U

V

W

Z